DR QUIN
MEDICINE MAN

DR QUIN
MEDICINE MAN

JOHN QUIN

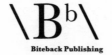

Biteback Publishing

First published in Great Britain in 2021 by
Biteback Publishing Ltd, London
Copyright © John Quin 2021

John Quin has asserted his right under the Copyright, Designs and Patents Act 1988
to be identified as the author of this work.

ISBN 978-1-78590-629-9

10 9 8 7 6 5 4 3 2 1

A CIP catalogue record for this book is available from the British Library.

Set in Minion Pro and Futura

Printed and bound in Great Britain by
CPI Group (UK) Ltd, Croydon CR0 4YY

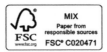

MIX
Paper from
responsible sources
FSC   FSC® C020471
www.fsc.org

For Maureen

'There are doctors who are craftsmen, who are politicians, who are laboratory researchers, who are ministers of mercy, who are businessmen, who are hypnotists etc. But there are also doctors who – like certain Master Mariners – want to experience all that is possible, who are driven by curiosity.'
– JOHN BERGER

"'I say, Doctor… this is no time to joke! Not at all!"
the general said to the doctor.
"Huh?"
"This is no time to joke around!"
"I'm not joking."'
– ANTON CHEKHOV

This book is a fictionalised memoir based on true stories, but many of the names have been changed to protect the individuals' privacy.

CONTENTS

PART ONE

SCOTLAND 1983–1992

1

COMEDIAN

He speaks softly to me with a gentle Dublin brogue. His lower lip is stained with a white smudge of Aludrox antacid that he takes for his chronic indigestion. He sits facing me in his neat office lined with leather-bound journals and the many PhDs he's supervised. I know that this man is the president of the British Society of Gastro-enterology and when I hear him tell me, with a calm insistence you might imagine he has when inserting a colonoscope, that I'm not a fucking comedian I near shit myself. You do not want to be faecally incontinent in the office of the country's top gastroenterologist. He has to put up with enough crap as it is.

The year is 1984 and I have been qualified to practise for just over eighteen months. I'm working on the South Side of Glasgow, where nobody seems to have ten fingers. The old boys that I look after have worked all their lives on the shipyards in the days when health and safety measures were, to understate the case, secondary to pro-duction. Two hours before the Irishman summoned me, he had sat with the other physicians watching as I presented a case at the grand round in the main lecture hall.

Grand rounds happen all over the country, usually weekly, and are a key educational opportunity for the medical staff. Rare conditions are sometimes presented, often in a teasing manner, with clues dropped here and there before, voila, like a magician producing the card you'd just thought of, the diagnosis is revealed and the case and its implications discussed. The presenting physician is the star of the show; he or she has to mug up on facts before the grilling that inevitably ensues from the audience. This is a test for young doctors: can they tell a story with skill, can they answer the quick-fire interrogation from their bosses, their peers? They are in competition with one another for references, for the next job, for a chance of becoming a consultant. I've worked on my turn for weeks. I know the timings, the gaps to get a laugh. I've played around with the lighting in the empty lecture hall the night before going on stage. I can do the talk in my sleep. The big day comes and I step up to the microphone.

Here's the punchline to my case. After the requisite details of the presenting complaint, the clinical findings on examination, the list of investigations, I reveal (because I'm secretly pleased to note no one in the audience has yet worked out the diagnosis) that we think the patient has... an amoebic abscess. I then say some more about amoebiasis that I have gleaned from the *Oxford Textbook of Medicine*, the big blue two-volume bible I owned in those pre-internet days. One detail about amoebic abscesses fascinates me: I learn that the pus looks like anchovy sauce.

Pathologists must have been a hungry lot in those far-off days when various medical conditions were first described. You can imagine them salivating as they hacked away at cadavers on those beautifully carved dissection tables in Bologna or wherever. See those they are teaching, tiers of them in training, looking down at the carnage below, all of them thinking about their next meal.

4

Pathologists talk of sago spleens and nutmeg livers. Pathologists are either starving or truly sick souls. I could never be a pathologist.

Back in 1984 I had never tasted anchovy sauce; I had never tasted an anchovy. This is Glasgow, you understand, before its famed Garden Festival, before it became Miles Better, before all those Turner Prize winners and the 'Glasgow Miracle'. But in the days leading up to my talk I knew what I would do in order to make my presentation memorable. I'd head to the supermarket. I'd buy some anchovy sauce. That, and a pan loaf.

At the highlight of my talk I took out the bread, whisked out the bottle of sauce and upended it so that the audience could watch the grey briny muck slowly ooze out over a fresh white slice. The smell was not good. But the stunt worked. I got a big laugh.

Then I slipped some other gags in, leaning forward to the mike, enjoying the amplified sound of my own delivery. This was a rush: I could see the grins, the smiles, and hear the occasional belly laugh. I was happy. This was being a doctor.

Half an hour later I'm back in the mess and sipping on a coffee, inwardly ecstatic at the hilarity I caused with my amoebic abscess success. I'm bleeped about an hour after my presentation and head to the phone. That soft Irish voice. *Could you come to my office just now, please?*

Everyone knew him as Gerry. Everyone knew that Gerry's uncle, or his great-uncle, was with Scott at the Antarctic. He leans back in his leather chair. 'That was brilliant.'

This is how he starts as I sit across from him in his office. He goes on: 'You paced that well, you got the main facts across, and you got a lot of laughs.'

He pauses and I thank him for the compliment, then he says: 'There's only one problem, though.'

A longer pause.

I wait and then he leans forward and glowers. His tone is urgent, insistent: '*You're not a fuckin' comedian.*'

Gerry's heart was in the right place, of course. The country's top gastroenterologist was widely regarded as both wise *and* hilarious. He could do fart gags during the many after-dinner speeches he was skilled at delivering. And he could play a mean fiddle. On ward rounds he would deliberately read the wiry squiggles of an electro-cardiogram tracing upside down and then pass them on to some underling, saying disingenuously: 'Tell me what this means, I've no idea.'

Years later I read a biography of Oliver St John Gogarty, and his character, his wit, powerfully reminded me of Gerry. Gerry was James Joyce's Buck Fucking Mulligan in the flesh. If said junior ostentatiously turned the ECG the right way up (and didn't get the gag) Gerry would be scathing a microsecond later. Behind their backs he'd turn to his trusted registrar and whisper: *prick.*

His idea of a weekend ward round was to sidle up to you in a corridor and ask anxiously: 'Everything's OK, yes?'

And then, when you said it was, he would thank Jesus and wipe once again at the white alkali stain on his chin, say cheerio and turn on his heels for home. This was his sign of trust. This was when you knew you were doing OK. If he had to actually *do* a ward round it was because he thought you were a prick.

Back in his office after telling me I'm not a fuckin' comedian he leans in towards me and explains. He stresses that you *can* get away with anchovy-related frivolity but only once you have established yourself, only once your colleagues have begun to take you *serious-ly*. I enjoyed hearing this paradox, but, perhaps noting my grin, he quickly pointed out that I was still a long way down the mine and could only act the goat, like him, once I'd made it: 'And that will take you about ten years.'

Ten years!

Maybe I'd been lucky to get even this far in the job. One of his colleagues on the north bank of the Clyde had told me six months earlier that my career in medicine was over. I was only four months into the career at that point. My sin? Mimicry.

His name was Hutchinson and he was a senior cardiologist and another renowned medical wit in the city. There was an ancient professor he had to work with, an uptight old guy. Hutchinson would point the professor out to us when he saw him lurking at the end of a corridor avoiding work. Hutchinson asked that we pay special attention to the professor's pristine white coat that he had buttoned right up to his Adam's apple. We would grin at this sartorial pomposity. Hutchinson had once told some wet junior, ignorant of the staff members, to go up to the professor and ask him if he could cut the hair of a patient in one of the bays: *he's the hospital barber, yes, him in the white coat over there, go on… ask him.*

Hutchinson was a bon viveur who would buy bottles of Pomerol for the cardiology team on their Christmas night out. He was well known too for his affected accent, this cultivated to disguise his more plebeian origins. He would lift his stethoscope from a patient's chest and ask me to go and have a listen in. Then the questions would start. Had I heard a third heart sound or a fourth heart sound on auscultation?

'OK, Quinnie, tell may, is thair a thid hot soind or aifort hot soind?'

If I said third he'd say fourth; if fourth he'd say third. I couldn't win. 'Care-dee-oh-loh-jay is not your fist soot, is it, Quinnie?'

I quickly mastered my impersonation of Hutchinson.

His manner was Olympian, but the supposed hot-air balloon of his ego could be exploded by the timely intervention of the notionally powerless. There was a well-known story of a toothless elderly patient from a rougher part of town who had once said to him, surrounded as he was by a large retinue of junior trainees, that she had known 'his maw, Maisie'. Maisie, maw of Hutchinson, had once been the old soul's neighbour and had lived 'up her close'. 'Close' being a narrow alleyway associated with slum tenements. The trainees listening to all this turned away to stifle their snobbish guffaws.

He once caught me laughing behind his back as he examined another lady's precordium with one hand while straightening his lank fringe with the other. He could see me giggling in the bedside mirror. *Calm yourself, Quinnie, I'm just adjusting my toupee.* One morning he called my friend and fellow house officer Ian McKay. The voice down the phone asked Ian: 'McKay! Where is that echocardiogram report?'

Eh-koh-care-dee-oh-grem.

Ian's reply?

'Fuck off, John.'

'Fuck off, John? That's an interesting reply, McKay. I take it you have concluded from our little exchange that I'm Quin?'

'Cut it out, John.'

The voice at the other end is now shouting at Ian: 'McKay! This really *is* Hutchinson! Get a hold of Quin and tell him to come up and see me right now! And tell him his career in medicine is over.'

I was twenty-two years old.

Mimicking a consultant. Biologists think, as with butterflies, that mimicry is a prime example of Darwinian evolutionary theory, a protective measure. By appearing to look like a leaf with grub-bored holes, the butterfly avoids being eaten by its predator. Maybe a cheeky junior doctor pretending to be a senior does not quite fit into this protective pattern; Hutchinson's tastes (I felt sure) ran to Chateaubriand with a Béarnaise sauce as opposed to tenderised slices of trainee doctor. With such childish behaviour I was truly acting like a junior. Maybe we were not evolving upwards as a profession. Maybe we were regressing. Certainly the persistent labelling of non-consultant doctors as 'juniors' was something many, particularly my father, would later regard as a prime example of medical infantilism. I can still hear him say, many years later: 'You're thirty years old! You're a senior registrar, for God's sake. How long are they going to call you a junior?'

Senior registrars, even if they were forty, were still 'juniors'.

I practised mimicry, honed my impersonations. The hospital had provided me with a small, lonely room in the liquorice allsort block of residences overlooking the M8. I would copy the traits of people like Hutchinson that I admired and then adapt them to my own fragile persona as a doctor.

Glasgow slang is called 'patter'. I was into thieving patter. It was patter theft. Even using this expression, *patter theft*, is stealing again. I stole it from a proper fuckin' comedian.

I stole stuff from all over the shop. 'Clerk-in' is the term we use for the process that begins with an introduction to a patient and ends with the documentary evidence of the encounter, currently on paper, soon (we keep being promised) to be electronic some time in the twenty-first century. Both the meeting and the document were termed thus: a clerk-in. I'd read and admired the various styles of clerk-ins and would rip off anything that took my fancy. I'd note presentational layouts that would call attention to the organised mind of the scribe. There were quirks in the calligraphy of some that would catch my eye, a tendency to higher legibility or a more extensive use of blocks, perhaps. Acronyms that I'd never come across could be particularly pleasing to pinch, such as PERLA: pupils equal and reactive to light and accommodation. This is a highly reassuring acronym to read; you do not want your pupils to be fixed and dilated. Problem lists at the end of a clerk-in made presentation easier when telling the tale to the consultant on (what we called in Glasgow) the post-receiving ward round.

In England, 'receiving' was known as the 'take'. Does that say something about the two cultures? One takes, the other receives? The 'take', then, was that group of patients we had admitted over the preceding twenty-four hours. I'd watch how my registrar bosses, Kris and Martin, would present information, how they would talk at meetings. I'd nick phrases from them that I found amusing because they would use them so often: 'Hi team!' or 'soooperb' or 'absolutely'. The game was then to sneak these into the conversation without them suspecting you were taking the piss.

I was reading Michael Herr's *Dispatches* at the time and, as the grunt on the wards, would do my best to try to squeeze some of that groovy 'Nam argot into the ward rounds. Coppola's *Apocalypse Now* was showing at the cinema. As the ward round started, Kris or Martin were in the Captain Willard role. This might begin with one of them saying to a group of house officers: 'Hi team, all set to roll?'

'Absolutely.'

'Who's in bed one?'

'Lady with pneumonia, she's on the mend.'

'And going home soon, I imagine?'

'Yes indeed, on Wednesday. Soooperb. Outstanding.'

Perhaps they might glower if your impersonation was a tad too obvious. As the years piled on, my patter on ward rounds became a palimpsest of gags and obscure verbal tics that were, in effect, the purloined references to people I'd long lost contact with and my current team had no knowledge of. And so all those words dropped randomly into ward conversations functioned as a belated tribute to all those who had trained me, even if the initial usage was only in jest. *Absolutely.*

Maybe this is true of all doctors: our style, like that of writers perhaps, can be compared to some glutinous smoothie drink concocted of various ingredients spun together in a blender before serving. You might sample one colleague's phrasing, his or her method of healthy exhortation as the spinach, the necessary green in the recipe; another's risqué gags might be the ginger, the spice. Whether the result, your style of bedside manner, was palatable would as often as not be a matter of taste.

Maybe Kris and Martin had seamlessly incorporated daft phrases from people *they* had once worked with and duly taken the piss out of, people from *their* pasts who had said 'hi team!', 'absolutely' 'seuntimetres' or 'soooperb' every two minutes or so. Maybe the kids *I've* trained over the past thirty years are saying these very phrases on the wards right this minute. Fuckin' A.

I'd even covet some highly stylised physical characteristics of my colleagues. I'd watch their gesturing as closely as one of those TV impersonators like Mike Yarwood who were all the rage in those days. I'd stand at the microphone in an empty lecture theatre before the audience arrived and practise copying a chopping gesture to emphasise a point that I'd learned from studying one of the brightest young professors in the UK. I'd yarwood a two-handed slow chop at the exact moment, at precisely the key point I wanted to stress. I was signalling that this, *this* (chop movement), was the take-home message.

My incessant parroting would become truly ludicrous in time. I remember much later in my career sitting in a management meeting that was predominantly staffed by male colleagues. The ape-like alpha power play committee nonsense was beginning to bore me. I studied the gestures around the table: the hands clasped behind the head pose that enabled the bearer to proudly reveal a damp patch of axillary sweat that stained his Jermyn Street shirt (a disgusting circular burst of rose on pink); the balancing of a prognathic chin on a thenar eminence as with the classic author pose. I decided to go the full Michael Corleone: arms and hands placed steadily on the wings of the chair, legs crossed at the knee with trousers hitched, the steely gaze held steady at the room. The gaze intended to be read by the others as hinting: 'I might go to the bathroom in a second to recover my revolver from the back of a cistern.' Amazing what you can come up with in order to get through a tedious afternoon.

Eventually such practised mimicry would extend to me pacing across a stage while lecturing. I'd imitate those monstrous egomaniacs who have colonised American medical presentations. I'd break up a pointless walkabout with an occasional insouciant lean on the lectern, again in the style of those Midwestern narcissists. While prancing about thus I'd tell the students that this style of presenting was precisely how *not* to lecture. This silliness kept them awake for five minutes before they resumed mutual relief in the back rows or whatever students get up to nowadays to distract their brains from Twitter and mountainous debts.

But I'd never master the impersonation of another American, one academic star who impressed me deeply. I came across this guy at an international conference on diabetes. His technique, hard won I suspect, was to commence a vague train of thought that would slow down as if his brain were a local steam engine approaching a minor country halt with a single platform. His logic seemed to be on a go-slow; it was as if he might (shockingly) grind to a halt with an appalled wheeze. But then suddenly, as if out of nowhere, he would shovel another spade-full of coal into the tender of his mind. His thinking would then fire up quickly and stun the audience with the gleaming terminus of his theory, his cathedral of cleverness: an Antwerp, a Milan, a Grand Central Station of a conclusion. Such an electrified high wire of an act would prove utterly beyond my mimetic abilities.

Some time in my first week working as a doctor I began a shift in the Accident and Emergency department, Casualty, or *Casuality* as the locals called it. The building was low-ceilinged and on one floor; the main entrance was on busy Castle Street, a road that connected the centre of the city to the motorway linking us to the capital and south to England. Ambulances queued up under a flat-roofed entry bay to empty their loads. A plaque to Joseph Lister hinted that this was a place of some seriousness; Lister came up with the idea of sterile surgery here. His was probably the last clean thought in the vicinity.

Across the road was the Manx bar, patronised by alcoholics with open tuberculosis. They drank beer and purple Buckfast fortified wine, spat gobbets of infected sputum onto the sawdust covering the floor. A+E was cramped and had many wooden cubicles, most open to the corridors, smelling of wet socks, pus and whisky breath. The place was once painted white but now had the yellowed look of old foxed paperback pages. A+E itself was foxed with brown spots of dubious origin. Privacy was a joke. The doctor's office was an alcove maybe ten feet by five feet in size, with shelves on high where you could grab a paperback formulary to check on drug dosages or score some spare sheets of paper. There were two or three phones constantly ringing: if you picked one up it might be the cardiology registrar who would maybe, just maybe, agree to come down and see someone who was worrying you.

Nurses wore paper hats back then with a thin coloured band that indicated their rank. A large woman with a green stripe that meant she was an enrolled nurse shouted at me: 'Room Nine, physician.'

I stared at her blankly. She shouted the same phrase again, if anything more insistently: 'ROOM NINE, PHYSICIAN!'

Again I looked at her stupidly, uncomprehendingly. Then she grabbed me and pushed me past the office and some limping souls on crutches and marched me to the far end of the department, where there was a stark room with no windows and one bed smack in the centre of the room, a room filled with scary equipment, a room that reeked of phenol. So this was Room Nine: the famed resuscitation room. A middle-aged man on a trolley was writhing around in distress and clutching at his chest. He looked pale and sweaty. My throat dried up. There were many other people in the room, some other nurses, this time with thick sky-blue bands on their paper caps; these were the more skilled staff nurses. There were ECG technicians too and a fat Shakespearean porter for comic relief.

I looked around at the stacks of shelves that held clear bags of intravenous fluid, pre-loaded syringes filled with lignocaine and other anti-arrhythmics. I sensed a deep well of expectation arising from all the others in the room now staring at me. Their faces sang in community and read the same message: *do something*!

I tried talking to the man, but it was no use: he was clearly incapacitated by his pain. Somebody (probably the big enrolled woman with the green-striped cap) barked at me: '*Should we put out a call?*'

A call? A call meant phoning switchboard to ask for the cardiac arrest team. I found my head nodding quickly in assent. The arrest team duly arrived in a panicked rush and eased me out the way and thumped on the man's chest.

And the guy? Well, he then promptly sat up and told them all to fuck off.

He was a regular. I learned this about fifteen minutes later from Mrs Enrolled with the green stripe. He was a timewaster, a chancer. He got his kicks by putting on regular dramatic performances in the various casualty departments of the city. I caught my breath and slumped into one of the three seats in the 'office'. Mrs Enrolled glowered at me. Her look asked: why hadn't I seen through his ruse? *Can't you spot a timewaster?* But then… why hadn't she?

Yes! Why didn't she tell me that as she shoved me into Room Nine? This I never worked out. A+E was my 'Nam right enough; A+E was *the shit*, my real dose of Michael Herr. The great William McIlvanney would later immortalise Room Nine in one of his brilliant detective stories. I knew within one week of my 'Nam, within one week of starting work as a grunt, that surviving A+E meant one thing: that I'd better get my shit together. Help was at hand.

Big Pat was a veteran GP trainee; he had the stare. Maybe not the fabled thousand-yard stare: let's call it the par three 150-yard version. He was a long-term resident of A+E and he consoled me – *you'll get used to it*. Big Pat was our enforcer. Pat and his mate Big Tom. Anyone over six foot tall in Glasgow is Big and gets called 'The Big Man'. You need Big Men in A+E. If there was any trouble with one of the more violent neds it would be Pat or Tom who would help silence them.

Neds. Folk etymology has this acronym standing for 'non-educated delinquent'. A ned would arrive at A+E and be placed in a cubicle. The screens would be drawn. This is how Tom would introduce himself to a ned pitching up after a sword fight: 'Ma name's Tom Madine, Mad Madine to you, and you can get tae fuck.'

And then the ned would politely sign themselves out.

Pat was quieter in his approach but was no less effective. Neds had 'chibs' (knives); neds were up for a 'square go' (ruck). You'd hear them swearing loudly, issuing drunken threats, more often than not with a sectarian tang, and then you'd hear the swish of a screen being pulled, some muffled scuffling and then… silence. Pat would emerge from behind the green drapes and look around to see if anyone was watching. He'd push the thick bridge of his glasses above his nose then head to Room Nine or our corner booth. A blue-striped staff nurse would then enter the cubicle with a sheet of paper. The miscreant promptly signed this: he was 'signing himself out'. The ned would then sneak out the department before being arrested.

Triage at the Glasgow Royal Infirmary was fascinating. There were three wooden boxes attached to a wall near our wee bothy, our wee wooden booth. The doctors squashed themselves up against the walls scribbling their entries into first drafts of clerk-ins. As they did this, the porters would pop buff cards containing one-line summaries of the new cases, or the GP's letter, into these boxes. The porters would meet the sick, the drunk, the abusive, at the front entrance and read the GP's letter; it was they who decided if the card they filled out should go into the left-hand box for the attention of the physicians, the middle box for the gynaecologists, or the right-hand box for the surgeons.

The physicians' box would be almost always full of cards. You'd dip your hand into the box like picking a card from a deck held out by a magician. Every case was a surprise choice! You might be dealt a juicy king, a case of *Legionella* perhaps, then much in the news.

Or you could land the nine of diamonds: a jakey with a trench foot crawling with maggots. Why the nine of diamonds? Said playing card is known as the Curse of Scotland – and one dark night we got a pack full of them.

Glasgow has had a gang problem for years, razor boys like the Tongs and the Fleet. There's maybe a hundred or more with daft names like the Sighthill Mafia, the Young Shettleston Tigers, the Carmyle Tahiti. Back in the '80s the top gangster was Arthur Thompson. He might nail you to a floor. Drug rivalries made the city ripe for turf wars.

The Doyle family came in as a group package after their house was firebombed. This was part of an ongoing gang feud now known as the Ice Cream Wars, a conflict that arose from local heroin sales. Ice cream vans would ramble around the meaner estates selling 99s, ice cream cones embedded with pillars of chocolate flake. But they'd also sell you a few bags of skag and a yellow plastic 'sin bin' full of used needles nicked from the hospital. The director of *Gregory's Girl*, Bill Forsyth, made a movie that chimed with the madness. He named the picture (with dark irony) *Comfort and Joy*.

I arrive for the morning shift just after 7 a.m. to carnage. What were white coats on the backs of my colleagues are now black rags stained with soot. Most of the Doyle family would die of smoke inhalation. Maybe about five of them made it to A+E first before succumbing in ITU. I meet my friend Eddie at the handover as we swap shifts, his face smeared with black stains. He looks shell-shocked, exhausted, his pupils large, his sleepless eyes heavy: 'It wouldn't have been so bad but we had to repeat lots of the bloods. We filled out the forms saying here's blood from a Mr J. Doyle. But then we realised they were called Jim and Johnny and Joe. And so we had to do them all over again.'

Some nights I'd cross the car park in the dark and get back to my room in the residences around two in the morning and play 'Sons of Pioneers' by Japan and stare out at the empty M8 with its flashing yellow signs warning of ice, its slick surface brightly lit by the overhead gantries. *Sons of pioneers, the hungry men.* I thought of myself as one of those hungry men, hungry for action. One month in country and I was getting used to it, getting into it. Being in A+E felt similar to being in the jungle under fire. I saw Big Pat as another Martin Sheen figure, another Captain Willard who had been in firefights, had run point more times than he could care to mention. Pat was the guy who shouts: 'Fire in the hole!'

And me? I was more like that wired know-nothing teenager from some South Bronx shithole. I came from a slightly tamer variant of the Wild West known as Westwood, East Kilbride: a 'new' town famed for its roundabouts. Polo mint city.

One night the following week I looked out at the motorway and its shadows and felt the early hours drag by. Watching the occasional lonely car zip west through the rain, I knew I should try to sleep but my mind kept going over and over the craziness I'd seen earlier that day. There had been another fire in the city. A wee girl of seven came in with 80 per cent burns, a sight I'd never want to see again.

A+E was my war zone and the trips down there were an adrenalised high away from the steadiness of my ward, my boat if you like. I'd have that line of Captain Willard's buzzing in my head every time I'd escape the hole, the hell of Casuality and get back to the wards or my kip overlooking the motorway, my hootch: *never get out of the boat.* I resolved to spend as much time as I could on my own boat: the ward in the block high above A+E.

A+E was like the sea, unimaginable in its fury at times. John Berger compares a doctor's role to that of one of Joseph Conrad's Master

Mariners. But I could see how as a mariner you could become lost and desensitised, and I got a sense of how you could even become despairing, become like Tom, or like Pat, thrashing out. Ultimately you might become a total degenerate like Colonel Kurtz, a Harold Shipman figure deciding arbitrarily who would live and who would die.

I would not become a consultant A+E doctor.

That kid, that wee girl. What had I just seen? Something I'd never visualised before and hoped I would never see again. But I've never been able to forget her image. What I saw was seared into my brain. When we see something horrific (something we've never come across even in photographic reproduction or TV or the movies) the retina receives the image and relays it the brain, where we try to make sense of what has just happened. But I couldn't make sense of this: not at first.

I'm standing in one of those jaundiced corridors of A+E about to clerk someone in. I've got my paperwork in my hands. And then there is a palpable sense of fear. People are running. Then she swept past me on a trolley fast on her way to Room Nine and the paediatric resuscitation team. There was a frantic air, a buzz of panic, and a sudden pallor in the faces of those who would try to save her. I saw the scarlet anger of her injuries. Both of her legs were bright red, this I remember. More of those black soot stains too that reminded me of the Doyle family, stains on her arms, stains on the white sheets. Even now I realise that I have been suppressing something. This is how we deal with true horror. How we try to forget the truly awful detail. But now I remember it all. The red colour was her legs and it extended upwards; the red line stopped on her tummy. I saw something you should never see. And I knew she would die. Here was a child in great suffering. And me? I stood paralysed in uncontrolled pity.

I knew now too that I could never become a paediatrician.

But A+E was, in many ways, less of a Coppola madhouse, and much more like a Mike Leigh movie: a Mike Leigh movie starring some of the saddest dafties on the planet. Bampots like those vacant-faced junkies who injected their femoral arteries with temazepam. They would then look down in appalled wonder at the mottled, marbled, pre-gangrenous appearance of their leg and say: *aye, just lap it aff, Doctor.*

There was too, this being Glasgow, the quick Stanley knife violence following the football that recalled the visions of another British film director, Alan Clarke, and his movie *The Firm*. And there were sword fights. Even doctors themselves were not immune to the dubious glamour of street fighting. Two of my colleagues came up to A+E following the sectarian madness of a particularly vicious Celtic versus Rangers game, striped scarves dangling from their wrists as they pinched their bleeding noses. Just another Saturday.

Sometimes one of the porters would sneak up on us quietly, touch our arms gently and ask if we could follow them outside. The white doors at the back of an ambulance would be opened and then we were ushered inside. *DOA*. If a patient was a DOA we had to climb up in order to certify the poor soul as deceased. This was done to prevent a fruitless dash to Room Nine.

I remember one freezing wet evening in January 1984. I stepped over some frozen puddles and was beckoned by the driver to clamber into the back of the fridge-like space where a shape lay on a stretcher. She was tiny and pale and very cold to the touch. She wore a thin blue-checked anorak and her hood was zipped up. She looked about seventy, but the driver said she was probably only forty-something. He knew her: she was a drinker, a regular over the road at the Manx, a regular too in A+E when she had had too much whisky. The sour smell filled the cramped space. She had no pulse and her pupils were fixed and dilated as I shone my pocket torch over her waxen, xanthic face. And I felt that controlled sense of pity again, a sense I would get to know only too well, one that I could maybe manage, one that did not make me want to crawl into a corner and shed hot tears as I did not long after seeing that doomed child.

That sour booze smell: my wife hates it too. A cabinet in our kitchen today is full of unopened bottles of whisky. These are presents, gifts for my retirement, from way too generous patients. Beautiful cylindrical packages. Three white boxes of Laphroaig. Some more yellow boxes of Glenmorangie, a solo bright-blue Talisker, an olive-green case with a 21-year aged Old Pulteney. I didn't have the heart to tell all those kind people this: I rarely drink the stuff.

I started working for the NHS at the beginning of August 1983. I read online, more than thirty-three years later, that on 8 September 1983, private contractors were allowed to tender for the cleaning, catering and laundering services. A man called Norman Fowler thought that this move would save up to £180 million a year. And no doubt he implied that this would be redirected to clinical services. And then a man called Ron Keating said that the move was 'a sword of Damocles hanging over 250,000 support jobs in the NHS'. As if the world needed more swords at the Glasgow Royal Infirmary.

In the beginning was my end. The slow process of privatisation had begun.

2

BLOOD AND GUTS NEAR
THE HIGH STREET

What made you want to become a doctor?
Every medic gets asked that: most have a quick reply.
Some hesitate. A minority of unfortunates are bullied into the profession by their parents for reasons of prestige or because the parents themselves were doctors. In time, the coerced become deeply
unhappy; they would have had better lives if they had listened to
their own inner ambitions.

It's a question that's difficult to answer truthfully: *why did you
want to become a doctor?* The response might be prompt but off pat.
The reasoning is frequently both simple – *I want to care for people,
I want them to get better* – and complex. This complexity may relate
to personal circumstance: there are many dermatologists who remember their own excruciating teenage years struggling with acne;
there are many oncologists with family histories of cancer.

So why did I want to become a doctor?

I had memories of visiting my Aunt June as she recovered from
open-heart surgery. I must have been nine or ten years old; she was

in her early thirties. She was in the Royal Infirmary: an enormously intimidating building across from the Necropolis, the grand ceme-tery high on a steep hill where the Victorian physicians of the city presumably buried their failures. June had rheumatic heart disease. When she was growing up in the 1950s rheumatic fever was not uncommon. Billy Fury and Andy Warhol had it. Andy developed something called Sydenham's chorea as a result of his rheumatic fever. This causes twitching movements, rapid jerkings, and was also known as St Vitus's Dance. Even now as I write I can hear Lou Reed's voice in *sprechgesang* going on about Andy making paper cats called Sam when he had St Vitus's Dance, in the album he did with John Cale about Warhol called *Songs for Drella*.

When I was young my mum would sometimes tell me to sit still when I was fidgeting and say: 'Stop that. Anyone would think you had St Vitus's Dance.'

I didn't know what she was on about and wondered if St Vitus's Dance was something like the bopping I had seen on *Top of the Pops*. I used to impersonate Mick Jagger, mimicry at age eight, and ask her (as I flapped my arms and pushed out my lips) if this was anything like the St Vitus's Dance.

June needed new heart valves. Now aged ten, I read everything I could about these valves in an encyclopaedia my grandparents owned. They called it 'The Blood Book' because it had a dark crimson binding. The mitral valve, the aortic valve, both with their cusps. Cusps like those small paper umbrellas (stuck amidst the ice in fancy cocktail drinks) I'd seen photos of in the Sunday papers. Cusps and chordae: thin wisps of thread that emerge from a small detail of anatomy I learned in time to be called the papillary muscle. Later, as a student, I would learn that patients with rheumatic heart disease could be recognised from the end of the bed because they had something called a malar flush; their cheeks stained bright red as if rubbed by excess rouge, a damson smudge a bit like the stain a cricket ball makes on a pair of white flannels.

And then much later still, in 2016, I was shown a monochrome photograph of June, taken around 1969, about the same time I was jaggering. Her cheeks are indeed dark smudges, that malar flush, markings as fateful as Stevenson's black spot.

I saw her last on 9/11 of all days. She was in her early fifties by then and those metal and plastic valves she'd had implanted were failing. She'd had at least three open-heart operations and there was no option now for another. She had developed pulmonary hypertension: a generally irreversible situation where not enough oxygenated blood gets around the body. She had ascites, fluid accumulation in her belly, and she joked that she looked as if she were heavily pregnant, as if she were nearly at term. This hurt her to say and it hurt me too as I knew she couldn't have children. She couldn't because she needed warfarin to prevent her getting a clot in her faulty heart.

Warfarin is an anti-coagulant, but warfarin is also teratogenic – it can harm a foetus – and so warfarin and pregnancy are a bad combination. Warfarin is *verboten*, contraindicated, a word I would get to know well. She next joked that she was now on Viagra, then under trial for pulmonary hypertension. She laughed and said: 'It's a bit too late now for any of that!'

I can see her grinning at the irony of her swollen abdomen, of taking drugs for an erection. Her face was tired and drawn, but her eyes still shone. The sun of her malar flush had now set. Dying, she still managed to express deep shock and sympathy at the horror of those images on the TV screen, the towers collapsing.

'Here,' she would say, 'do you remember when we would get bottles of ginger from the Alpine van? American cream soda and some vanilla ice cream, a 99?'

That stick of chocolate flake she loved. This would have been thirty years before her final days in hospital when her parents, my grandparents, were alive and when she had fallen pregnant. My grandparents on my mother's side (strict Catholics) had eight children. Ken Dodd once joked 'a stitch in time saved nine', but vasectomy was not an option for Papa, my grandfather. June had fallen pregnant in her early twenties; she was advised not to continue her pregnancy: *the warfarin, you see, it can damage the baby.*

Now she looks away from the Twin Towers falling and asks me, with her eyes gleaming: 'They will forgive me, won't they?'

They: she means what she understands to be those at the Higher Court. She means St Peter. She means Jesus Christ.

Her parents, my maternal grandparents: I remember when I was in my teens talking, shyly, to my grandfather about love. He was a sceptic. When my grandmother walked into the room I said: 'Well, you love Nana, don't you?'

And without missing a beat he pointed to his wife and said: 'Her? *Love her?*'

She looks at him in distaste and he continues: 'I love Rangers more than I love her.'

I think I remember him grinning. And what of my own parents? They did not put me under any academic pressure; they did not suggest that I become a doctor. They loved music. And music would infiltrate my whole world, my thinking, even if I could never play a note. I have an expressive deficiency, a minor parietal lobe malfunction, I assume. This means I struggle to coordinate my hands, *ma hauns*, with my brain. I'm what Glaswegians call *haunless*. But my receptivity for music is reasonably acute. I find it hard to avoid referencing what I like hearing. My dad played piano at home: 'Moonlight Sonata' would make my mum cry for a bit, but then he'd play some boogie-woogie that he'd learned doing National Service, which would cheer her up. My mum is very sensitive to music too and her eyes would well up listening to the *Carousel* soundtrack. Gordon MacRae musing about becoming a father, his putative baby boy Bill, or would it be a girl? Gordon realising he's making all these plans and his kid ain't even been born yet. My mum could never listen to 'River Deep – Mountain High' after she had a stillbirth in 1966. My dead brother, Peter. Even now, when I hear those ominous opening chords I think of her. And him. Her thinking about him every time she hears the dread first lines: *When I was a little girl, I had a rag doll.*

My parents encouraged learning, bought me a book I liked on marine biology when I was ten. I particularly liked a photograph of a manta ray that a shark had been munching on; the semi-circular chunk out of a wing looked like a bite out of a sandwich. And then there were the corals: brain coral with its convoluted sulci, and the colours, the colours: electric blues, gaudy pinks. Maybe I could become a marine biologist. But I was, and remain, a rubbish swimmer.

I should have worked out that it was the colours that really attracted me. This love for colours and pictures that would make a lot more sense to me later.

Mum and Dad liked to watch *M*A*S*H*, the TV series, though Dad might have seen the film version too because he used to be a regular at the Glasgow Film Theatre in the 1960s. Dad was an

Altman kind of guy, relaxed, another sceptic, fond of a cigar and a glass of Bell's, often screamingly funny. He would make jokes at Mass on Sundays. When the priest told us to 'make the sign of peace' my dad would flash a hippy V-sign, or he would whisper 'gie's peace'. He knew his Nouvelle Vague: *The 400 Blows* was one of his favourite movies. And neo-realism too: he loved *Bicycle Thieves*. I can picture him getting upset at the scene where the young boy discovers that his father has been arrested. I think it made *him* think that this must never happen to us. His own father had died when he was fourteen, so he had no father figure then. He had to make it all up.

All I know about my paternal grandfather is that he served in the First World War as a bantam, a wee guy, somewhere between four foot ten and five foot three inches tall, leading ponies up to the front with ammunition. He did this for four years. Mad. When he returned, he got political, became a Conservative. How does that work?

I assume he rejected John Maclean and the nascent Glasgow Soviet. Maybe Granddad was a kind of midget Ernst Jünger reactionary figure allied to some crazy Glaswegian version of the Freikorps. He had books by Quintin Hogg, another Tory. I remember that book on his shelves because of the absurd forename. How could you have a first name that sounded like a surname? There's something oddly Scottish about this combo. William Boyd often names his characters like this: Lorimer Black, Logan Mountstuart. But my grandfather had nothing in his shelves about the First World War, no accounts of blood and guts, nothing by Jünger: no *Storm of Steel*, not that I remember.

In the 1930s I think he might have been an appeaser, at least at first. Many men who survived the First World War were. This is hard for people to understand now, but then we've not spent four years stuck in the mud with only a pony and the bodies of your dead friends for company.

Anyway, we watched *M*A*S*H* together as a family. And I liked Hawkeye: Alan Alda. I thought that a life in medicine might be like the world of Hawkeye Pierce. Entering my teens, I imagined myself wearing greens stained with blood, cracking gags with the nurses. All the nurses (bar Hot Lips Houlihan) seemed to like Hawkeye. He got laughs, he got girls, and he got covered in the blood of brave soldiers. He was a good guy; I wanted to be like Hawkeye. He was a comedian. What a ludicrous advert for a life in medicine. But I bought it.

We were hauled up for a careers talk when we were aged thirteen. I told my teacher that I wanted to be a doctor, but I didn't talk about Hawkeye. This was my Latin teacher, Mr McVittie, who also doubled as the career adviser. He told me to drop Latin and I remember being impressed by this: he'd told me to reject the very subject that he taught. How cool was that? But his reasoning was sound. You didn't need Latin to study medicine in this day and age. There were no patients in Glasgow called Davus or Flavia or whatever... so Latin was out. Art too, he insisted. You don't need art to get into medical school. Colours would have to wait. Art wasn't greatly encouraged in the East Kilbride of the early 1970s.

So in time I applied for medical school. Now, years later, in this twenty-first century, I'm watching Bobby Gillespie from Primal Scream on the iPlayer and he's saying that if you were from Glasgow in the 1970s you could only escape the drudgery of the workplace if you were good at football or if you joined a band. Bobby and the rock 'n' roll mythos: he had also been in the Jesus and Mary Chain, who were also from East Kilbride. But what if you were unmusical, crap at football *and* had a vestigial parietal lobe?

You could be a swot on the sly. I filled out the forms for medical school when I was fifteen and got accepted. Sounds crazy but you could do that in Scotland. They told me that I should do a sixth year at high school first (*take Higher Spanish, it'll do you good*) and then go up to uni when I had turned seventeen. I dogged school and hung around the countryside in a place called the Glen drinking cans of McEwan's. In cavalier fashion I failed the Spanish. *¡Sinvergüenza!*

Learning this and sensing I wasn't cut out for a Mediterranean existence, my parents promptly left me. I was sixteen and they took my brothers and sister away for a new life in Malta with its sun and rocky beaches, its *passeggiata*, its baked pasta and fizzy Cisk lager, leaving me to five years of Glasgow in the driving rain and cold. They were beaming as they waved bye-bye at the airport. The Britain of bin strikes and Jim Callaghan and the decaying prog rock of Emerson, Lake & Palmer were now behind them. *Enjoy your studying.*

Five years later, elsewhere on the Med (in the October of that first year as a doctor in 1983) came news from Beirut that a truck bomb had killed over 200 US Marines. But this was only one of the very many horror stories that had been coming out of Lebanon at that time: the kidnappings, the massacres in the camps. Beirut was the last place on earth I, or anyone else in Britain, wanted to visit. In 1983 I would not have believed that Beirut would play a happy part in my future.

Oddly I heard recently from a friend telling me that one of the surgical wards in our local hospital is jokingly known as 'Beirut'. This I did not know. Beirut is where patients with cirrhosis are admitted. This is particularly the case if those unfortunates have tortuous varicose veins sited at the bottom of their gullets, known as varices. These can suddenly rupture. These, no other word will do, *geyser* blood. They shower everyone within fifteen feet with buckets of wet, sticky blood. There are words that strike immediate fear in doctors. *Varices*: that's one of the worst.

Variceal bleeding. In those early days of my working in the NHS, getting an endoscopist to inject the veins with a sclerosant – stuff that makes them shrink – was not easy. There weren't that many gastroenterologists: maybe two per teaching hospital, one if you were in a district general. To temporise we would be told to stick something called a Sengstaken tube down the patient's throat. This recalls Vladimir Nabokov's frightful memory of 'controlled panic' when he was confronted with a bronchoscope. He described the scope as a 'vulcanised rubber tube'. Controlled panic and a recipro-cal controlled pity on our part: the relationship between patient and doctor simplified.

A Sengstaken tube is a thick rubber affair (imagine a garden hose with inflatable balloons attached to one end and plastic entry por-tals at the other) into which you inject some water. The water blows up said balloons that can, in theory, compress the leaking veins. In theory. Trying to get an alcoholic, often violent and abusive (*fuckin' fuck off, ya fuckin' fucker*), or the drowsily encephalopathic (the brain swimming deliriously in a bath of non-metabolised am-monia) or a combination of all three to swallow said tube was, in Registrar Kris's words, 'character building'.

Trying to avoid being drenched in blood was nigh-on impossible. Tarantino's cinematic sanguinary excesses are thought exaggerated but they are for real when varices give it the full Old Faithful. A rite of passage for young doctors, then: the squelchy, sticky walk back to your flat to get changed. A stomping moonwalk as someone else's blood, the blood of a cirrhotic (maybe even Hepatitis B positive!) fills your pair of Marks & Spencer's brogues, the blood soaking through those white Paul Weller socks you'd proudly bought with your first pay cheque.

Beirut, the ward today: a Boschian hell of blood fountains. But Beirut the *actual* city would play a benign part in my life during the twilight of my career. My brother got married there and it was a strange experience to walk along the Corniche wearing a kilt; local families mobbed us to take a photograph with them. Fame at last. Fame with your only fans a handful of the Hezbollah. His wedding was a delight and I'm now a proud uncle, even if my fabby multi-lingual Arabic/German/English-speaking niece makes me feel as thick as mince.

Another reason to reject gastroenterology as a career, aside from frightful wrangling with the tentacles of various flexible scopes, was the stench. I was too fastidious. The seniors made us do rigid sigmoidoscopies back then, meaning a cold stainless-steel tube inserted up your anus. Then we would have to document how many centimetres we had ascended to. Fifteen centimetres, twenty-five centimetres. As a student I was assigned to work with a pretentious surgeon who pronounced the word *saunt-eh-maitres*. And he had a gold-plated stethoscope. A surgeon with a stethoscope. That's a workable definition of a poseur.

There were a few quite bizarre consultants working in the early 1980s. This minority, then nearing retirement, really thought they were gods; that society owed them big style for reluctantly agreeing to work for the NHS after the war, for accepting that stuffed mouthful of gold from Nye Bevan. They were a different breed: a different class. They were *above*.

But in reality, gastroenterologists are very much below. They are down below with their sigmoidoscopes. You would smear some lubricant and then stick this steel pole up and under, then, bending, squint at the view that would be pink or scarlet. The stink was mighty. How could gastroenterologists do this sort of thing daily, hourly?

Bleeding at the top end of your guts eventually comes out the other end as melaena. Melaena is not some forgotten Greek actress but the term for black tarry stools that suggest significant upper gastrointestinal bleeding. And melaena has a distinctively horrendous smell, a rotting sweet aroma that turns the stomach. You can detect it quickly on entering wards like Beirut. If you wish to experience it yourself without real risk then I suggest a meal of three or four slices of Stornoway black pudding. Warning: avoid any interaction whatsoever with other humans for at least forty-eight hours. Melaena is another gut reaction word in medicine.

Enough gastroenterology. Ward work at the Glasgow Royal Infirmary as a junior house officer (JHOs: the lowest of the low) meant a daily morning round with one of the consultants. Invariably the JHO pushed the trolley full of notes like a bored shopper in a supermarket while listening obsequiously to pearls of wisdom from the master. The boss would hear out your one-minute reminder of who the man in bed twelve was, then have a brief chat with the patient, and then come up with a plan of attack for investigation and management. On the days that our team was in charge of any new admissions, the JHO would visit A+E and do the first meeting and assessment of a patient: this was that 'clerk-in' I mentioned. We would later present the case to the consultant on the 'post-receiving' ward round.

This presentation was greeted by them in a different manner of styles: usually with respect but sometimes with a barely disguised tone of sarcasm. Tales of humiliation on post-receiving ward rounds would be swapped around the JHOs when we would get a time-out for coffee. We heard of one unfortunate who had written in the notes (as a concluding diagnosis) the phrase 'triple vision'. The game for physicians was to suggest the most outlandish diagnosis to the consultant, and extra points were earned if the conclusion turned out to be accurate. We each had our successes that we might brag about over games of Donkey Kong in the mess. They had a doctors' mess in those days. And in England at that time many hospitals even had a bar that would fill after shift's end.

My one real success in presentation on a post-receiving ward round involved telling the consultant about a young girl who had arrived in A+E with a fall after a seizure. I asked for her calcium level to be measured and it was in her boots. We X-rayed her skull and noted extraneous white markings that suggested she had some calcification in the brain. I looked at her hands and saw, oddly, that she had an absent knuckle. Proudly I wrote my first proper diagnosis in the case notes: *Impression: 1. Pseudo-hypoparathyroidism.*

I waited impatiently for the ward round and then said, with a quietly restrained flourish, that I thought the girl might have pseudo-hypoparathyroidism. The consultant, the boss, a Professor Fraser, leered over the top of his spectacles: 'JDQ... are you sure you mean pseudo-hypoparathyroidism and not pseudo-pseudohypoparathyroidism?'

He was fond of referring to colleagues by their three initials. His were JBF. Later, over coffee, he sensed my disappointment that I had not quite impressed him as much as I'd hoped. He warned me with a sigh: 'JDQ, don't get your bowels in an uproar.'

Flash forward to 2016 and my bowels are most definitely in an uproar. I'm having a screening sigmoidoscopy (clinical science now suggests that this might save lives) and I'm curled up on a table while a young woman sticks the tube up me. 'We'll get it to about fifty centimetres.' *Fifty centimetres!* I'm relieved to hear her pronounce it *sent-uh-meetres* and not *saunt-eh-maitres*. The tubes are flexible now. I can see the folds of my colon on the TV screen above my head; a pink tunnel that I pray will not reveal an obstruction, a polyp, a cancer. Her assistants have the radio on and are trying to calm me by talking about the DJ and his choice of songs. Don McLean is singing about Vincent and that starry, starry night.

Van Gogh spoiled for ever.

3

THE ROYAL

B ack then junior doctors were given an on-call room. We did overnight stints after a full day's work, shifts that exceeded twenty-four hours. The longest uninterrupted stretch I worked was from a Friday morning starting at 8 a.m. finishing on the following Monday evening at 5 p.m. A grand total of eighty-one hours on duty. In fact, we did this not infrequently, maybe about twenty times that first year. Nowadays newly qualified doctors rarely get a room or a bed because their shifts are much shorter. Their workload, however, is intense; medicine can do a lot more good.

Our residences were in a building that looked like one of those black and white striped liquorice allsorts. The architect had probably been to Florence once and, excited, thought: *Right, I'll do something inspired by the Baptistery.* Maybe he guessed it would make a bright contrast to the imposing shadow of the Red Road flats. These eight multi-storeys (each with twenty-eight floors) looked like a dystopian archetype, a nightmare vision straight out of a J. G. Ballard novel. The residences looked like the Baptistery if you were high on a cocktail of temazepam and Buckfast. They sat squat alongside the stream of traffic on the M8. Trying to sleep there during the daytime with the flatulent wheeze of artics braking under the gantries was a challenge. At night you could hypnotically watch two rivers of light in motion: one in red, the other in white. Pretty.

Putting lots of young people on shift work in one building was, of course, a recipe for much hanky-panky. A few off-duty nurses would stand and talk and smoke and flirt outside the residences well into the early hours. A fire alarm went off one night and it was faithfully reported that one of the housemen had to be uncuffed from a bed by the firemen. Frankie Goes to Hollywood's 'Relax' was the big hit and the mess parties had a suitably debauched flavour. The song seemed to upset a few people at the time, the prudish disc jockey Mike Read for one. As if DJs back then were exemplars of moral authority...

At the same time, Davy Henderson from an Edinburgh band called Win sang: *There's no more protection, it's a highway of infection.* HIV was not really an issue in Glasgow, 1983. Wasn't that some strange illness gay people were getting out in San Francisco? We only knew one guy in our year who had come out.

I remember reading the first paper on AIDS in the *New England Journal of Medicine*: the abstract talked about men who had an average annual number of partners of just over 1,000. Like most people just out of their teens, we thought: *No one has a thousand partners a year, do they?* Nah, surely not. Talking about the paper around coffee, we guessed this must be a misprint. No one had a clue what it all meant. The disease also seemed to affect Haitians for some reason, but all I knew about Haiti was Papa Doc, Graham Greene's *The Comedians* and voodoo. Voodoo and zombies; none of us planned a trip. Didn't Papa Doc once have a fresh corpse propped up against a wall at Port au Prince Airport with a sign around its neck reading

'Welcome to Haiti'? Years later I came across a paper in the *British Medical Journal* about zombification in Haiti. Zombies actually exist.

I'd finish a night shift then head down to the city centre like a zombie myself (a pseudo-zombie or a pseudo-pseudo-zombie) and pass the urban campus of Strathclyde University. I'd then take a left to admire the giant protractor-like glass and iron Victorian immensity of Queen Street Station. I liked to walk across the statue-infested expanse of George Square, thinly populated at this time in the morning, and head to a place called New York, New York, where I'd order a burger and fries and a beer. This was before 10 a.m.; the streets now quiet as the commuters settled at their desks. Maybe I'd also get a slice of cheesecake. I felt like Travis Bickle in that scene in *Taxi Driver* where he sits in a downtown diner numbly staring into a cup of coffee. *I'll work anytime, anyplace.* I'd go through my memories of the previous night's encounters with the traumatised, wiping blood off a couch in A+E just like Travis does with the back seats of his cab.

The blood was my fault. I'd been trying to stick a Venflon in the arm of a drunk. Venflons were the plastic cannulae we used to hitch people up to IV fluids. We fetishised Venflons because they came in different bores and these were colour coded by their small caps, the portals where you stuck a syringe filled with diuretic or antibiotics. The pinks were slim, ideal for kids with thin wee veins. Green were standard issue and grey were large-bore, ideal for running in blood quickly (*stat!*) if someone needed a transfusion. These grey ones were stuck into the cirrhotics in case their varices went all Etna, the full Stromboli, on us. We considered it cool if you could get a grey Venflon into someone with poor veins. Kris was universally admired as the King of Venflons.

Past midnight A+E was full of the freaks. They'd all come out at night. Was (Not Was) had a song back then with a chorus that ran constantly around my head as I sat with my burger in New York, New York thinking about the previous night on call I'd survived. *Woodwork squeaks and out come the freaks.* I'd finish my chocolate fudge sundae and trudge back to the Baptistery residences for a kip.

I'd pass the crumbling soot-stained Victorian brownstones of the old Merchant City, throwbacks to a more affluent era, the time of shipbuilding, of Burrell and his ilk, Burrell with his bulk-buying of art treasures. Much of this old money was obtained from the slave trade: hence Jamaica Street, Virginia Street. Streets named after those tobacco lords like John Glassford. There's debate now about renaming some of these streets; maybe they should. There are plenty of better candidates for remembrance, like the city's great scientists, artists and writers. Comedians, even. We should have Connolly Street, Limond Boulevard. Or better still McCune Smith Street. James McCune Smith, born a slave, graduated from Glasgow in 1837 at the top of his class; he was the first African American to receive a medical degree. Crowds greeted him on his arrival back home in New York City. New York, New York. I read recently that Glasgow University has agreed to pay £20 million in reparations to the University of the West Indies.

Film directors often use Glasgow as a location mimicking New York; a scene from another Batman movie is currently being filmed up at the Necropolis. Back in the early '80s many of these architectural gems awaited reappraisal and not a few were neglected; some even had trees and shrubs sprouting on high from the top floors.

Sticking my paws deep into the pockets of my sodden cagoule, I'd dip my head as the rain slammed down then trudge up the High Street. The road curved upwards to the hospital and was peopled by the city's unfortunates, jakeys with their carry-oot. They slugged on blue-black bottles of lurid yellow-labelled Buckfast. The road climbed up to the fortress on Castle Street, the black soot-stained gothic immensity known as the Royal Infirmary. I was certain I would meet some of those drunks again tonight in A+E. Drowsy as a result of all that American stodge, I reached the residences, alone, unready for another overnight shift.

The hospital, the castle, was a massive Victorian pile with crenellations and ramparts and might even have had a moat somewhere. There were cupolas and a clock tower; the overall effect had something of Mervyn Peake's *Gormenghast* about it, or Kafka's castle. The Kafkaesque problem about the Royal was not that you couldn't get in: it was that you had a hell of a job getting out. I was still regularly clocking in over a hundred hours a week.

The place was enormous. There was a modern extension that housed part of the medical school. The whole edifice sat smack bang in the historical centre of the city. St Mungo himself was said to once dwell here, long before the Manx bar and A+E. Glasgow's odd mythology about a fish with a ring in its mouth saving the Queen of Strathclyde from certain death apparently began on this spot. From most of the medical wards where I worked you had a view of a hill where the city greats were buried: the aforementioned Necropolis, a testament to the vast wealth the city had extorted through the exploitation of slaves.

The Necropolis was a maze of baroque dark mausoleums the like of which I'd not see again until a visit to the Recoleta Cemetery in Buenos Aires when I was in my fifties. Our patients in the Royal could sit up in their beds and stare out at this city of the dead and contemplate their ending, all our endings. And they could listen too, every summer, as the marching bands (the Orange Lodge or the Irish Republicans) banged their drums and blew on their flutes as they passed below. The sectarian hordes would head up Castle Street, some no doubt ducking into the Manx to get stoked up before a sword fight and another trip to A+E.

Imagine yourself dying, knowing that you are *actually* dying. You're stuck in a bed in the castle, the Royal, and the last sounds you will ever hear are the thumping booms of the big drum, the tunes of division; a soundtrack of hatred for people like you, Catholic or Protestant. This was the reality for some of the people I cared for. The city fathers are not keen on banning these processions of bigotry. In 2020, in a gesture of supreme sacrifice, marches were cancelled in the face of Covid-19.

The transport people apparently argued for years as to whether Glasgow's buses should be painted an Irish-referencing green, white and gold or plain old Protestant orange. I heard a popular rumour that this oft-changing decision reflected the numerical divide amongst the elect at the City Chambers.

A priest once told me that he paid a visit to an old lady on the ward who was dying and he tried to comfort her with kind words. 'I'm fine, Father,' she told him. 'I just stare out the window here and see thon beautiful tall tower on the brow of the Necropolis and thank God that the statue of Our Lady is looking down on me.' He hadn't the heart to tell her that she was looking at a 200-foot-tall memorial topped with a stone carving of John Knox, the father of Scottish Protestantism.

The Royal was wedged between the motorway, the Necropolis and the fearsome rectitude of the cathedral. This gothic house of God was consecrated as far back as 1197 and is named after St Kentigern, confusingly St Mungo's *other* name. (St Serf is said to have given Mungo his pet name.) The streetlights around the cathedral have a carved feature representing Mungo's miracles. This is the city's coat of arms: the tree that never grew, the bird that never flew, the fish that never swam, the bell that never rang. Mungo brought a dead robin back to life: that bit I remember. This scene is now depicted on a terrific High Street tenement mural.

Across from the cathedral sits the Provand's Lordship, the city's oldest house, a place that none of us had ever visited. At the back of the Necropolis there was a brewery and the Wills cigarette factory. Ghosts might wander around the monuments of the cemetery looking down on the city. From on high they could neatly map out their former lives as a mini-odyssey. A tight orbit that encompassed places where first they poisoned themselves with booze and fags. Then it was over to the church, where they prayed for health. Next it was a mere pop across the road to the hospital. Here they sickened and died and were lastly carried up the hill to be buried. It's a great view.

Below the wards in the Royal was an extensive network of underground passageways, a maze of interconnecting subterranean corridors, a cramped, dank place with metallic tubing on the ceilings – ventilation ducts, I assumed. And there were wires running parallel with the ducts and some loose ends dangled here and there, the arteries and veins of the building, you might say, supplying power to the operating theatres. The tunnels made an immediate impression on the imagination, a chthonic world with strange inhabitants. Unsurprisingly a real writer would latch onto this place: they are referred to in Alasdair Gray's magnificent Lanark. One can make a strong argument that Lanark is the novel of the Royal Infirmary. Poor young asthmatic Alasdair spent more than his fair share of time stuck in the Royal; as an old man he had another extended stay after a bad fall.

Down in the tunnels we would scurry with request forms for radiology: scan asks. Computerised tomography (CT) was a new technology then and you had to individually discuss these asks with a consultant radiologist. This involved embellishments, exaggerations, to get what your consultant wanted for a patient: *yes, his pupils are unequal.* The radiologists sat in tiny offices and listened with ill-concealed boredom. They would nod cynically and sometimes agree to the request or, in pique, send you back under the pipes to the lifts for another quizzing of your boss, who in turn redoubled your mounting irritation, the frustration of it all.

I did not want to become a radiologist.

If the lifts were not working it was a slog up the solid foot-worn stone steps and back to the ward round. I worked on Wards Four and Five. These were Nightingale wards, with the nurses' station at the top end with views down to the two rows of beds. Single-sex wards were scrupulously maintained in those days, Ward Four being female; Five, male. The consultant I'm working with grabs the trolley of notes and off we go. He writes in the notes. Most consultants do that here in Scotland, this is the norm, and I'm struck years later at the inability of many of my southern English colleagues to do the same. An oddly instantaneous dysgraphia comes upon them whenever they are presented with a case. *I can't quite seem to grasp this writing lark.* Is this a parietal lobe problem? The seniors in England use the juniors to 'scribe'. They say they have not enough time to write. Maybe this is something to do with flunkeys, a distant nostalgia for the colonial life. Or maybe it's a canny defence in court: *I never said that!*

There is an elderly woman in the third bed, a Mrs Bond. She has picked on my boss. Like some dreaded equatorial parasite, like

Onchocerca volvulus perhaps, she has insinuated herself under Dr Hastie's skin. She has chronic pain but no sinister pathology. There is more than a suspicion that she is 'at it'. At it? *It?* The 'it' means swinging the lead. A timewaster. Her manner is wheedling, whiny. She has written to my consultant weekly for many years now. Over coffee he has read some of her letters out loud to the team. She calls him 'the son of the devil'. Dr Hastie, in actuality, is a true son of the manse.

He laughs as he reads them out to us, but he's upset. Dr Hastie is a quietly religious man: he's from the Outer Hebrides and they hold God and the Sabbath very dear up there. The devil is not some abstract concept for the Wee Frees, those who worship God at the Free Church of Scotland. Up there they have no sympathy for the devil. Up there Mick Jagger *is* the devil.

I can tell that Mrs Bond does not impress Dr Hastie; I can tell that he is offended. *Very* offended. But I also know he can be a very funny man; he has timing. He really is a fine comedian. He buttons his white coat up tightly and has bottle-lensed glasses that he takes on and off during the round. He removes a (correcting) red pen from a top pocket to scrawl in the notes. He spends an age over the first patient and then tires as the round progresses, his natural enthusiasm now spent. He somehow contrives to escape Mrs Bond, a quick nod to her and he's on to the next patient. But she's on to him: 'What do you expect me to do, Dr Hastie?'

He ignores her because she keeps telling him he is the son of the devil. This happens twice more that week: *What do you expect me to do, Dr Hastie?* On the following Monday he is refreshed, he is ready for her. He introduces himself: 'Hello, Mrs Bond, how are you today?'

Her reply is sullen and clipped: 'How am I today? TODAY? What do you care? What do you expect me to do?'

He tries his best to mollify her, but she drones away like a washing machine; she is indifferent to the real suffering going on in the surrounding beds. She loves the sound of her own voice: 'But what do you expect me to do, Dr Hastie, what do you expect me to do?'

He looks up at the ceiling in despair.

Her needling voice again: *What do you expect me to do?*

He turns to me, leans nearer my ear and says this quietly in his best Sean Connery accent: 'I expect you to die, Mrs Bond.'

I convulse. I gasp. I have to leave the ward right now. Outside I fall in the corridor and I'm literally rolling around in laughter. *I eggshpect you to die.* When I return Mrs Bond calls me over and asks me if I'm all right.

'He's the son of the devil that Dr Hastie, you know that, don't you?'

Dr Hastie. His first name was Sinclair. Apparently a character in one of the bestselling fictional books about doctors popular in the 1960s is based on him as a junior. Crazy Sinclair. I'd know if I'd pissed him off because he would call me 'son'. I'd maybe forget what someone's potassium level was. Tempted to say four – aim for the middle, I'd think – but then my conscience would kick in and like Washington I'd resist the lie and admit that I didn't know.

Look, son.

Days off would see me out walking again, my cagoule hood up against the drizzle, walking without direction around the city centre. I'd dream of the many other cities I'd never been to. Various landmarks were architecturally reminiscent of buildings I'd seen in books. Some of the buildings on Argyle Street had Swiss gables, another looked vaguely like something super-functional from the Bauhaus. There was the Templeton carpet factory, styled after the

Doge's Palace, and the Waterstones bookstore near Central Station, inspired by that other Venetian masterpiece, the Ca' d'Oro. Persisting with the Italian influence, there was also that dark medieval Bolognese tower where they used to hang criminals, the Tolbooth Steeple, still standing at Glasgow Cross.

Many, many years later I'd explore the vibrant gallery scene on nearby Osborne Street and drink in the 13th Note and Mono with its murals by Lucy McKenzie. In the early '80s this area was ill lit: a dead zone of pubs catering for those unhappy souls drifting up to the Barras, a cheap market, in search of a bargain. Some places around here were notorious. The Saracen's Head, a pub known to Robert Burns, and known to all as the Sarry Heid, was reputed to sell 'the Blue Monkey'. I never dared ask for a glass. The Blue Monkey was methylated spirits, meths. The real drinkers here made Malcolm Lowry look like a zealot for the Temperance movement. Bobbing and weaving on their way home, you would catch yourself swerving out of their way.

One night my wife and I watched one tall member of the species swing back and forth on his heels near the Saltmarket only to fall solidly onto the pavement like a felled sequoia. I can still hear his head crash as it hit the ground. We were on our way to the Barrowland ballroom to see a band from Northern Ireland called That Petrol Emotion and already somewhat wired that trouble might lie ahead given the band's known Republican stance and the sectarian nature of bars in the area.

I felt for his pulse: nothing. He wasn't breathing. His face looked lined: he might be in his seventies. Which probably meant he was about thirty. I raised my fist and thumped it down on his chest, aware of how drastic this might appear to the connoisseurs of violence inhabiting these parts. My wife did the mouth to mouth: a moment that still turns her stomach given the foul stench of blended whisky. We got an ambulance, we got him to A+E, and then we got cheek from the admitting team, our colleagues: *What are you guys doing? Touting for business?*

We learned the next day that he had died. A massive stroke.

'You look so young, Doctor, so young.'

If I heard that phrase once back then I heard it a thousand times. Actually this is from Bulgakov's short story 'The Towel with a Cockerel Motif'. And maybe I did look like the kid I really was. Maybe I was just a boy. Like the young Russian doctor, I used to lie in bed when I was on call and try to imagine what I might have to deal with that night. This was a superstitious rite. I figured that if I thought of a scenario, thought through how I would act, then perhaps it might never happen. Magical thinking. I'd go through the various medical emergencies and visualise how I would proceed if, for example, someone came in with a pneumothorax (a collapsed lung) or a haematemesis (vomiting blood) or a pneumothorax *and* a haematemesis. I saw medicine as a multifaceted Rubik's Cube, each face of a cube being a diagnosis, each face of the cube an unpredictable, near-random, combination of diseases. As I began to drift into sleep, the scenarios became ever more baroque until my fears would peak with that classic medical horror story: a pregnant woman having a cardiac arrest. What the hell would you do faced with a pregnant woman whose heart has stopped?

I'd picture myself cutting open her stretched belly and hauling out a flaccid green and brown meconium-stained baby. Meconium is that shitty stuff that surrounds a babe in trouble, a word my wife, a delivery suite sister, liked to use a lot years later when I was eating my evening meal. Picture it: big plate of spag bol, fork laden, mouth open, saliva flowing, and then hearing a senior midwife say that word out loud. *Meconium.*

Lying in bed I'd visualise the next step in my gruesome scenario. I'd then have to open up the chest of the pregnant woman (a gleaming set of silver chest cutters to open up her chest – *fuck*) and then lean in to compress her stilled red heart and... and... and... then BLEEP-BLEEP-BLEEP, my page would go off in *real* life now, now I'm wide awake, and I'd jump out of bed knowing that it would be the dreaded call to the obstetric ward but no, no, no... it would be a voice on the phone asking: 'Could you come and see Mrs Clarke, the old lady in bed eighteen, she's fallen and we think she's OK but we think you need to come and check her over. It's policy. Sorry, Doctor.'

Actually the bleeps do not go BLEEP-BLEEP-BLEEP. It's a much more annoying sound, an incessant EEEE-EEEE-EEEE, a high-pitched mosquito whine that you cannot sleep through, that you cannot swat, a buzzing annoyance, a screaming fire alarm of a noise that will stay in your head for ever. EEEE-EEEE-EEEE in the early hours usually translates as *you are wanted right now because we are in big trouble.*

Another day at work, the patients bled, the ward round done. Venesection was crucial, phlebotomists were not employed back then, and so we would be on the wards at 6 a.m. to puncture the arms presented to us. *Is this for the black pudding factory, Doctor?* We'd have the trays with the equipment set up the night before, the syringes in their blue and white packs, the green plastic guarded needles, the different-coloured bottles for the blood: pink-topped for haematology to get a haemoglobin reading, plain white for biochemistry to get the electrolytes. Setting this up was the last job of the day before leaving the ward for the Manx and its beer, its sawdust, its tubercular customers.

One test we would have to do daily was something called the erythrocyte sedimentation rate, the ESR. Purple-topped bottles if I recall. The ESR is a useful catch-all, a simple test that allows physicians to know if something drastic like serious inflammation or metastatic cancer is going on. A normal value does not exclude such fears but makes them less likely. So the bosses would ask for these on most of our bed-bound souls. Each small purple-topped bottle that we had filled with blood could be placed on a special rack and into each we would then place a thin plastic tube, not unlike a thermometer. The idea was that we would watch the rate of fall in the level of blood down the tube in one hour: the faster the fall, the higher the ESR, the more we worried.

But how to get the blood sucked up the tube in the first place? Well, there was a rubber sucker we were supposed to use, but we could never find it. And so we would line these tubes up, maybe twenty or so in a row, and then lean over each one, purse our lips and suck on the top of the tube with one eye on the rising column of blood. We would stop sucking when the blood reached the top. Except that sometimes you would get distracted or harassed, *There's a radiologist on the phone wants to speak to you*, and you would suck a little bit too powerfully and get a lukewarm mouthful of blood. There was then an instantaneous nausea and that familiar rusty iron taste and a fast rush to a tap to rinse as much as you could out of your mouth and clear it all away.

Simultaneously over in Atlanta, Georgia, the Centers for Disease Control and Prevention, the CDC, were increasingly sure that the cause of AIDS was… a blood-borne virus. The warning went out. Avoid contact with infected bodily fluids. Right. I can't remember there being a new batch of rubber suckers arriving for us after this breakthrough.

The fast bleep goes off, a faster frequency EEEE-EEEE-EEEE than the usual call to arms, and this more frantic sonic attack implies that someone is having a cardiac arrest somewhere. Miraculously, a voice from switchboard comes from the bleep telling us which ward to run to. The arrest bleep always comes as a surprise; it's like some malcontent creeping up behind you only to thump you on the back of the neck. Like the man said about your own death, you never know the hour. In fact, it dawns on me that the arrest bleep goes off precisely when you least want it to, when you delude yourself that you've got things in control. In control! Tip for young doctors: you are never in control.

I wish I'd known this as a young man: there's no point being a control freak because the random chaos of life on this planet is the norm. But by the time you really learn and understand this you have already become the kind of obsessively controlling fusspot that cannot leave a house without checking the doors and windows and taps and grill and plugs and doors again. And then the windows a second go, just in case. And then the doors, one last time. Some doctors develop a full-on obsessive-compulsive disorder that requires psychiatric help. Problem is that to some extent the public expects doctors to have some mystical control over natural events: our fault I guess for raising expectations, for daring to take on fate.

You cannot get on top of the inherently chaotic, as with someone's heart that has an ejection fraction (a piece of medical jargon that says what it means on the tin) of less than 20 per cent. Just when you think you have everything sussed the world goes EEEE-EEEE-EEEE. Then there is the lurch in the stomach, the rapid rush of stress hormones from your adrenal glands, and you are off and running, pelting down empty sickly lit jaundice-coloured corridors, jumping downstairs five at a time.

One night I heard the slapping flap, flap, flap of feet belonging to a cardiologist as he ran barefoot to an asystolic person on whom I'd already began cardiac massage. After attending your first few arrests you realise that the chances of success are very poor indeed, that you are coming in at the end of the game. The ones that survive cardiac arrests are generally on the coronary care unit. Here on-tap cardiologists and nurses shock the patient out of some dysrhythmia consequent to their myocardial infarction. The ones *we* got called to were the elderly with pulmonary emboli, huge clots that blocked the blood getting to the lungs for oxygen, and these commonly happened when the patient was on the toilet seat. Evelyn Waugh apparently died in this manner.

And so a gang of us would arrive, breathless ourselves, and invade the cramped lavatory. We'd drag the body into some space with elbow room and thump on the chest and charge up the defibrillator. This made a spooky *zeeeee* sound. Someone would shout loudly before the electricity was applied, *SHOCKING*, and we'd all stand back. Two hundred volts and the patient would jerk like a giant puppet. Then we would have some more chest pummelling applied by some rugby-playing junior. And lastly a senior person (huffing and puffing) would arrive at the end of the bed and would work out that all was in vain and call a halt. Cardiac arrests are pretty awful.

On one occasion I was called to an arrest with my friend Danvers, who was training in cardiology at that time. In between compressions I looked up at him. He decided to have a go at an intra-cardiac injection of adrenaline. This he did in advance of the notorious *Pulp Fiction* junkie scene with Uma Thurman. Danvers had done it many times before. A nurse handed him a loaded syringe and with a thrust he punctured the chest wall. From the top end of the patient came a dull Edinburgh drawl that announced with some sarcasm: 'That's not where the heart is.'

Danvers ignored him. The Morningside bore tried again: 'THAT'S NOT WHERE THE HEART IS.'

I look up at this east coast anaesthetist bagging at the top of our motley tableaux, a balding man with a bland butter-coloured ball of a face. His knuckles whiten as he compresses the black bag in a vain attempt to oxygenate the poor pale body on the bed. Danvers withdraws his syringe filled with pillar-box red fluid (he's in the heart for sure!) and stares up at the gasman. I've never seen Danvers look this way before: he is the most benign of men and is usually close to infective hysterics of laughter about some absurdity, but he is snarling now, his teeth bared, his eyes beaming with malice. We're losing the patient big style and I decide to call it a day and then tug Danvers into a side room before he explodes: he is for thumping the anaesthetist. He calms down over a cup of tea.

That's what happens in medicine: you calm down over a cup of tea. *You'd like a cup of tea?* Your mind is yelling out: no, no, I don't, I do not want a fucking cup of tea, not now, not ever, because a cup of tea will not bring my patient back! And yet you accept a mug. Moral of this tale: never *ever* tell a cardiologist where the heart is.

But where is the heart? Maybe the great writers know. Some say James Kelman might. Some say James Kelman should win the Nobel Prize. I'm doing some rewriting just now and take a bit of time out to look at Twitter and read a tweet from a journalist called Rebecca Myers who is based in Glasgow. She's got an article in *The Times* today about Kelman, who admits he hasn't voted in nearly fifty years. Hasn't. Voted. Fifty years. The article is titled by a phrase he uses in the interview: 'We turn away from suffering and avoid reality.' I can hear all those who have worked in Scottish medicine these past fifty years wanting to say this to him: James, *you* might have been tempted to turn away from suffering and avoid reality in the voting booth but that's not an option for those of us working in the NHS.

We learned very early on as JHOs that you could switch your bleep on and off with a great deal of ease. There was a small knob that you pressed to the right, click. You're now off. And then you could press it back to the left and EEEE-EEEE-EEEE, you're back on again. This was particularly useful during dull grand rounds when you could bleep yourself out and head for a sleep-postponing coffee. I quickly understood why doctors drank so much coffee: it was either that or inconvenient bouts of narcolepsy, your face falling into a bowl of canteen soup. So you would switch the bleep off and then on again for the gizmo to send out its irritatingly loud three-bar trill.

The more daring, carefree juniors would do this trick in order to pop out for a cigarette halfway through one of the more boring consultants' ward rounds. As with those in particular featuring one Dr Douglas Anderson, a pinched, hunched-over figure with cadaveric features and a droning, one-note vocal delivery. What was it with certain senior Glasgow medics who assumed these monotonous tones? I suspect they reckoned that it gave them gravitas: the whole point was to appear unenthusiastic, to affect a 'seen it all before' bravura. Mind you, Anderson would think nothing of starting an undignified public spat with a colleague over their rota, much to our voyeuristic enjoyment. He usually lost these battles, as his challenger was no less a figure than the president of the local Royal College, a man much venerated as a skilled clinician. I'd have my own discomforting situation with the president later.

The bleep could be misused in other ways. You could ask

switchboard to buzz a colleague for, say, the boiler room. Said colleague would come back into the mess puzzled and wonder: 'The boiler room? Who the hell wants me in the boiler room?'

A teasing gang crowding around that Donkey Kong machine in the mess would titter.

Or the bleep could mimic other functions. One notorious GP trainee was said to own a pair of joke spectacles that he would produce if anyone pestering him in A+E asked what their chest X-ray looked like. He'd pull the dark pair of shades out one of his pockets, slip them on and then tell the patient what he saw. *Looks clear to me.* But on one occasion a mother could not be placated so easily. Her child had banged his head and she was insistent: 'He needs a CAT scan, Doctor.'

The GP trainee shook his head: 'I don't think so. Look, he's fine, see? He's smiling at me.'

Mum's face reddens and she raises her voice: 'Ahm tellin' ye, he needs a CAT scan!'

'No, look, c'mon, he's running around, he's fine, just a little concussion, that's all.'

'He needs a fuckin' CAT scan, Doctor! Dae it. Dae it now!'

And so the GP trainee put his hand down and switched his bleep off and then on again. Next he pulled the bleep out of his pocket and then the mum watched him as he waved it like a wand over her child's head while the little black box made its squeaking EEEE-EEEE-EEEE sound. The child was transfixed. The GP trainee stared at his bleep with exaggerated concentration and then looked up at the mother and concluded: 'See! Nae problem. CAT scan normal.'

I can't even tie my shoelaces properly and so it was clear to me, even as a student, that I would not end up as skilled as Hawkeye from *M*A*S*H*.

I would not be a surgeon. I would not spend most of my day prancing around in greens cracking the funnies to a bevvy of admiring nurses as he did. In time I would (unbelievably) perform an appendicectomy with a senior surgeon known to all as Gorgeous George, but I'd like to offer belated apologies to the person whose abdomen I entered with a scalpel. I'm sure your scar should have been a lot smaller.

Surgeons went on about yachting and rugby and looked at you a little oddly if you said you spent your spare time reading. The physicians, though, well, they went to see plays, art exhibitions. They were the chin-strokers of medicine. Physicians stood at the end of the bed and listened very carefully to a patient and heard their story and then they thought for a bit. And then thought for a bit more. A hand would come up and a chin would be stroked. (A carefully shaven chin. I have known only a few physicians with beards. One grew a beard because when he shaved it off he looked about twelve years old. I remember talking to him years later about how good Joy Division were back in 1979 and he looked at me like I was mad. I think he was in his mid-fifties back in 1979.) And now in the twenty-first century the bookshops are full of bloodthirsty autobiographies written by... surgeons. How in hell did *that* happen? Since when did surgeons become so literate?

There was a TV cigar advert once, maybe for Hamlets, which claimed something like 'I've never had to make a decision I couldn't take half an hour over'. That was being a physician. You generally had a bit of time to mull things over, sometimes for an age. Physicians like to mull. Physicians would mull all day long about anything if you let them. They'd mull about mulling. They'd mull about a holiday on Mull. They'd mull about the wisdom of mulling about a holiday in Mull. And they liked signs, clinical signs.

Signs! Semiotics. I liked *actual* signs too, the physical ones. Those old blue British Rail signs. As a boy I'd nicked a giant THORNTON-HALL sign from an old signal box and stashed it in a wood. Too big to take it home. Then there were I-Spy books that made you look out for other signs. Those smaller red triangles on the roadside that you occasionally came across near a pier with a black car going over the edge into the sea, or those scary ones that just read '!' There's proper minimalism for you, a sign that says '!'

Clinical signs, though, well, they are like semiotics in action. I was becoming a physician.

Clinical signs are not really like semiotic signs; they are not a mere label for a thing like, say, the word 'girl' as Scritti Politti sang back in those days when I was first becoming sign-obsessed. No, clinical signs imply pathology. They are often non-specific: indeed, their usefulness is now being seriously challenged in these times of advanced MRI scanning. The Royal College of Physicians is even wondering now how much time we should spend on teaching the recognition of signs. But their presence can suggest a diagnosis *before* expensive tests confirm or deny a suspicion. And although we often have time to chin-stroke, every now and then something happens very quickly. We may not have time to wait for the result of the expensive test. This is when the presence, the detection, of signs can be valuable. These signs have wonderful names like:

1. Whispering pectoriloquy:
Here we listen to the chest with a stethoscope and ask the patient to whisper 'ninety-nine' in the time-ordered fashion. If the ninety-nine sounds coarse and high-pitched (imagine a hoarse German saying NEINTAY NEIN) then there may be an underlying pneumonia. And it looks very cool if you can demonstrate this to trainees *before* you get a chest X-ray confirming the diagnosis.

2. Shifting dullness:

Not an orthopaedic surgeon on the move, as the old joke has it. What happens is this: you are faced with a distended belly and you think it contains fluid. Fluid in the belly is called ascites, as with my Aunt June. You can pronounce this *ass–cite–ease* or *ass–kite–eez*. I've never worked out which one is correct. Maybe both are. And so you then percuss the abdomen. Percussing is that tapping business we do with one finger rapping on another. So we percuss the abdomen and then tilt the patient, all the while percussing and listening for a change in tone. If there is a lot of fluid on board then this shifts on tilting – the fluid *and* the percussing tone: hence shifting dullness.

Ascites is a usually a bad prognostic sign: we find it sometimes in patients with metastatic cancer and also in cases where excess fluid retention has occurred due to heart failure or cirrhosis. Most physicians have a sad tale where they have examined a young woman presenting with an abdominal swelling. The woman not unnaturally thinks that pregnancy is the likely cause. The pregnancy tests are found to be negative and the scans then discover that the real culprit is an ovarian cancer.

3. Chvostek's sign:

Endocrinologists love this one. We tap the cheek over the facial nerve and watch closely to see if the face then twitches. This implies a low calcium level. Again you can appear clever when about twenty minutes later the lab phones back with the result you have predicted.

4. Delayed reflexes:

A personal favourite. Ask the patient to kneel on a chair with their ankles protruding. Swiftly tap on the Achilles tendon with a tendon hammer. The ankle jerk, the reflex, is slower in its recovery phase than normal. This can be a sign of an underactive thyroid. I've seen generations of trainees and the odd professor of surgery stare in amazement as the ankle slowly jerks back. They are then duly shown the estimate level of thyroid-stimulating hormone from the pituitary gland that confirms the diagnosis of an underactive thyroid.

Physicians are commonly known as 'the magicians' by the other specialties in medicine because they think we deal in the fuzzier aspects of diagnosis. They think that being a physician smacks of quackery, of alchemy, of wizardry, wands, the use of strange potions. But they know too that it can imply just a hint of cleverness.

Physicians are into intellectual snobbery. *Go for it because that's what the clever doctors do.* I think someone might even have once said that to me. This might be the real reason I didn't go in for surgery or radiology or anaesthetics. I think I wanted to become a physician because that's what we were told the clever doctors did. That's what others of my ilk thought at the time too. It was cool to be a clever doctor, an expert. Not a rich one. But that was back then.

That first job spanned the autumn of 1983 to the spring of 1984 and involved a sequence of jobs on a rotation, beginning with Dr Hastie and his wanting to strap Mrs Bond to a metal table being bisected by a laser beam. This was a general medical ward. The specialty of the ward team was diabetes and I was quickly inducted into the mysteries of insulin and its dosages. 'Throw the bones up in the air and see how they land' was Dr Hastie's jokey response to my asking how much insulin we should give to a new patient. So it was informed guesswork then. Medicine can be an extremely empirical game to play.

Fear and panic were never far away on the wards, if not in such a frenetic manner as in A+E. One of my fellow naïfs couldn't take it. He was found hiding in a cupboard. He went on to study economics and is no doubt a far calmer and wealthier man today. One evening a nurse phoned me urgently. She was shaking when I arrived: an insulin pump had been wrongly set and a man had received fifty units of the stuff in half an hour, way above his usual requirement, way above anyone's usual intake. I called Kris the registrar and he asked me tersely: 'When was this noticed?'

I asked the nurse and she shouted over to me: 'About half an hour ago.'

Kris is then quick to ask: 'And he's all right?'

Again I mouth the question to the nurse, now biting her nails: 'Yes, he's fine. Blood sugar is six.'

I relay this back to Kris.

'Then you're OK, JDQ: insulin has an intravenous half-life of about five minutes. Relax.'

Calm reassurance was never a given.

4

WARD ROMANCE AND A
NASOGASTRIC TUBE

From the diabetes ward I rotated to a small rheumatology hospital that was off-site on Baird Street near the VD clinic. This was a five-minute walk away on the main route from the city centre to the central police station, an imposing block of rain-stained concrete at the foot of some sky-scraping council flats. I'm introduced to Janet, the senior registrar. She shook my hand and asked: 'So you're the new house dog?'

Next sentence she tells me to be careful as she's on her period. Will do. Three months into the job: Janet is my first female boss. She's as sharp as a scalpel and in time becomes a professor.

In the middle of one night on call at Baird Street I'm phoned by the sister in charge to deal with a man at the front door: 'Eh?'

'Can you come to the front door, please? There's a man here who insists that we let him in.'

Someone's knocking at the door. Do me a favour. I get out of bed, dress and go down the stairs to open the lock just as the man is about to hammer on the door again. He's a vagrant swaying with the whisky he's been slugging all day and he's after a room for the night. I tell him as politely as I can that this is not a hostel, there's always the Great Eastern, close the door and clamber back into bed. Ten minutes later I'm bleeped again to come down and write up a narcotic for an insomniac. Medicine: you get skilled at quickly putting your clothes off and on. Those dark early hours thinking ludicrously: *Should I put on my tie?*

Rheumatoid patients are in so much pain and I feel impotent in the face of their suffering. It will be many, many years before the breakthrough of the so-called disease-modifying drugs, which will transform rheumatology into a specialty that can actually *do* something for patients. Back in 1983 I decide against specialising in what seems to be a discipline with no future. Predicting the future in medicine is as difficult as any other form of speculative guessing.

After another month I was sent to a chest hospital a couple of miles away from base camp at the Royal. Here I would be shown how to stick drains into the chests of those highly unfortunate enough to have something called an empyema. An empyema is a collection of pus inside the chest. As I type, I can relive the experience of putting in my first drain for an empyema. Infiltrating the local anaesthetic, the wait until it takes effect, taking the needle out the pack. Taking the weapon, like a thick knitting needle, in my gloved hand and now pressing it against the muscle of the chest wall. And... *push!*

The ammoniacal stench as the pus was released literally knocked me off my feet. The waft of the smell hit me like a punch and I swayed, gagged and fell. I remember hitting the floor. I got up and wiped at my wet eyes then connected the plastic drain to a collecting bottle. Eyes still streaming, I sewed the drain into the skin. I watched the creamy goo of the custard-like pus slide down the drain into the glass bottle.

Chest medicine wasn't for me either.

That patient got better but there was a strange woman in the next bay who was in this chest hospital for ages. She would suddenly stop breathing for no apparent reason: an arrest call would be put out, EEEE-EEEE-EEEE, the team would arrive and thump at her chest and then, abracadabra, she'd sit up suddenly, now gasping for breath and that would be that. This happened so often over a period of some weeks, sometimes more than once a day, that we got used to getting called to see her for urgent resuscitation. One night she told me that her husband, a policeman, had seen some film footage of someone being killed.

I told the story to my new chest boss the next morning and he looked askance; he never mentioned the tale again. After another six or so 'respiratory arrests' I asked him the following week if she might have Ondine's curse. I didn't know what this was but had read about rare cases where the brain stops sending messages to the chest telling it to breathe. This was called Ondine's curse in the textbooks. Again the boss looked at me sceptically. *You're reading too much.* Wasn't Ondine someone at Andy Warhol's Factory? (No, he didn't ask me that.) The next day he called and wondered if I fancied a trip to London.

My parents had returned unexpectedly from Malta and now lived in Essex. Essex was a very different place from Glasgow in 1984. Even so, this was my chance to see them again. I leapt at the offer: 'Sure, I'd love to go. But why?'

Turns out the boss had phoned the Brompton, the UK's centre for unusual chest problems, and they had accepted the woman as a transfer but had asked for a doctor to accompany her. And so it was that I travelled down the motorway in the back of an ambulance for 500 miles with what might be a fantasist. I don't think the Brompton ever found out what was wrong with her. The psychiatrists assessed the woman and couldn't identify any mental health issue either. She was not a schizophrenic; she was not depressed. In plain language she was not thought to be mad or sad. Was she just *bad*? She had what physicians, with their coded language, call a 'functional' disorder. If you hear the word 'functional' when you see a doctor it probably means they think you are having them on.

Many of the patients in the chest hospital I worked in had end-stage chronic lung disease, or lung cancer from smoking. The place truly was the anteroom for death. Doctors like golfing analogies even if they rarely get a chance to play it this century. Well, the Grim Reaper was on the down stroke in that joint.

Decades later I'd read that a colleague in the year below me who also worked in the same chest hospital had died as a result of a mesothelioma, a rare tumour of the pleura, the lining of the chest cavity, caused by asbestos. A tragedy: I'm not sure if the doctor, who had a young family, even made fifty. That chest hospital we worked in was full of asbestos. You couldn't make it up. The local health authority admitted liability.

After a torrid month at the chest place I'm back at base camp, the diabetes ward in the Royal. I'm covering on the wards and it's been a quiet Saturday so far; all is calm. The sister phones: a lady has been transferred down from dermatology. She's stable but can I review her? Sure. A routine task. No problem. Half an hour later she phones again: 'That lady with SLE that I mentioned, well, she says she can't move her legs.'

'Her legs? Are you sure?'

'Yes. And I don't think she's having us on.' Sister thinks this is not 'functional'.

'When did this happen?'

'She says it only happened ten minutes ago, just after she got settled into her bed here.'

SLE (systemic lupus erythematosus) is a dread disease that we know all too little about. Essentially it is a vasculitis: the blood vessels are inflamed. And yes, that's 'lupus' as in wolf. You don't want a condition that has the word 'wolf' in its title. Didn't Hitler call himself 'Wolf'? I rush up and sure enough this lady, her cheeks reddened by a rash in the butterfly distribution classic of SLE, cannot move either leg. She can move her arms and trunk and head but… she cannot move her ankles, her knees, her hips. And she can't feel them either. Her circulation looks good, her foot pulses are present, the dorsalis pedis easily felt bounding ahead of her big toe. But she cannot feel me touching her shins. She has had an instantaneous paralysis in both her lower limbs and only now, as I examine her, does she show signs of fear. Something truly dreadful has happened to her.

Time to phone Kris the registrar again: the King of the Venflon. He listens to the story and knows what is going on here but, as a good teacher, asks me first: what do I think has happened? I hazard a guess that she may have infarcted her spinal cord. There is silence on the other end of the line. Maybe I'm being pretentious. Maybe I'm *havering* as we say in Glasgow. Waffling. I speak up: 'I think I read about that somewhere.' And then he's back quickly: 'Agreed. Good thinking, JDQ.'

Physicians, once respect has been accorded, once it is acknowledged that respect is due, seem to get called by their initials in the Royal: FSF, MCA, ACR. I think I might have just joined the club. He tells me to get her transferred to the neurosurgeons across the city. This means a tough negotiation with the neurosurgical registrar, the beginning of a mutually antagonistic relationship with those guys, one that has now lasted thirty-three years. They agree to take her and I'm appalled to hear later that Saturday evening she had a cardiac arrest on arrival and died.

At post-mortem she was found to have clotted off her artery of Adamkiewicz, the main artery supplying the spinal cord. She had infarcted her cord right enough. This is a very rare complication of SLE. Later I tell the story to Janet, the senior registrar in rheumatology from Baird Street. She's working on a new drug and says: 'You should have phoned me, we could have given her our new wonder drug, prostacyclin.'

Would it have been ethical to give the woman an untested drug in an emergency without even being sure of the diagnosis in those pre-MRI scanning days? Perhaps. But many back then would have said no, the majority probably. Who knows if this might have saved her? Maybe it would have. But what if it had gone wrong? Medicine is full of maybes. Dealing with uncertainty daily is draining.

Next month I'm back doing cardiology with Hutchinson: 'Oh, not you again, Quinnie!'

He points across the ward: 'Now go and listen to that man's heart over there and tell me if he has a third heart sound or a fourth heart sound.' *Soind*.

I belatedly gain his respect by calling a cardiology registrar at 3 a.m. when I realise that the second shot of frusemide I've given a man recovering from a heart attack hasn't improved his breathing. Frusemide is a diuretic and an incredibly useful drug at 3 a.m. if you are faced with a man in heart failure. But this guy is not winning. He's gasping for air. He's drowning in his own body fluids because his heart is not working as a pump the way it should do. His pump is a flabby, flaccid sack. I listen in to his chest, I auscultate. His lungs have what are known as 'fine crepitations' on auscultation. This sounds like the noise your hair makes if you rub some strands right in front of your eardrums.

Why was his pump failing? This is what you have to do in medicine: *ask the question*. Keep asking questions.

His heart attack was thought to be mild. I look at my notes. I've written that he has a systolic murmur. He has a whooshing noise in between his first and second heart sounds. I can't hear a third or a fourth sound, but then, as Hutchinson knew, I never could hear them anyway. But if *I* can hear a murmur then he definitely has one. I look at the older admission notes and they read: HS 1+2+0. Heart sounds one and two and *no* murmurs. This murmur is new. And then I think carefully. A systolic murmur that is now best heard under his armpit. My brain connects; I remember my teaching. This man has mitral regurgitation. This man has developed mitral regurgitation suddenly, acutely. And this must mean that he has ruptured his mitral valve. One of those papillary muscles has gone. I know this to be a rare complication of heart attacks. I know this too: he needs emergency cardiothoracic surgery like, like... like *now*! And he gets it. He lives. My Aunt June with her own faulty valves, her own knackered papillary muscles; Aunt June would have been proud of me.

After six months as a trainee physician I swap over to the surgical side to work with Professor Haig. He has white hair growing over his collar, a salt and pepper moustache and a calm, distinguished manner. He sits behind his desk about a mile away from the door to his office. In the background somewhere a tape machine is playing Gregorian chant. I walk in expecting St Peter to appear at my side, St Peter the Rock, wondering if I'm to be allowed entrance. I'm here to ask the prof., God, if I can get time off to have a cancer removed.

The timing is not good. One of the other housemen, Doddie Grieg, has taken time off too because he can't hack it and so I'm worried they'll make me stay on. The surgical senior registrar, a guy with a Zapata moustache, made me do the night on call after this Doddie Grieg punter phoned the registrar to say he was 'too tired to come in'. And Zapata spoke to me – no, ordered me – to do Doddie's shifts. That made me on a one in one. On call *every* night.

This madness lasted three nights until someone somewhere came to their senses and got a locum. This kind of thing would be a recurring theme in all my years as a doctor, asking people to cover illness. Latterly it was my task to find the locum, usually late on a Friday afternoon, to ensure the weekend was staffed appropriately.

God, Professor Haig, was a good guy and let me go and get my tumour cut out. Maybe I'd impressed him with that slow ankle jerk I'd demonstrated on our last ward round together. I'd seen his face light up as he watched my prowess with a tendon hammer. *See! This patient is hypothyroid.* He was thinking: *Maybe physicians have their uses after all.* The magicians.

I remember his face another time. We were in a lift together after one of his patients had just collapsed and died from a pulmonary embolism. The cardiac arrest team hadn't won. Professor Haig had removed the patient's primary liver cancer a few days before. He was sure he'd got it all out. The patient was forty-something. Professor Haig's face in the lift: grief-stricken. Grief about his patient and, too, grief over the fact he knew he had done a great job. He looked like the once omnipotent Marlon Brando in *The Godfather* after he's told that his eldest boy Sonny has been shot. God can be beaten.

The pathologists found I had a leiomyosarcoma on my arm. Another clinician and colleague, a good friend, urged me to get it seen to. I'm seriously in his debt. In time he would become the best man when I married.

The timing of the diagnosis was *really* not good. Cancer is not what you want to hear when you understand that you have fallen in love.

The surgeons I now worked with on Prof. Haig's unit were a classier bunch than I'd expected, some quoting Burns on ward rounds. Only one of them physically assaulted me: Zapata. I think he's now some big wig at the Department of Health. He picked me up by the lapels of my white coat, slammed me against a wall and asked me where in hell some barium enema report was. That Zapata moustache: how come some of the surgeons wore big bushy moustaches back then? Over in America the Village People were huge and having fun at the YMCA. The clone look was in at Studio 54, but I think tough Glasgow guys in scrubs packing knives weren't quite aware of all that. This was long before surgeons could write bestselling memoirs, of course.

I'd have to get up much earlier when I was doing my surgical job. Sometimes we worried about reeking of the pints we'd sunk about six hours before. We got started on the venesection, maybe as many as thirty patients to bleed, at six on the dot in darkness; the ward lights would only go on at seven. But by ten we were finished for the morning because surgical ward rounds did not involve chin-stroking. They comprised quick inspections of wounds and fluid charts and then the senior surgeons would make a dash to theatre. For us their escape to the operating table meant an early trip to the mess for a bit of Donkey Kong and some more nuisance bleeping of colleagues to say they were wanted in the laundry room or the GUM clinic or some other dubious venue.

The surgeons did encourage you to go with them to the operating room, but I'd had had enough of all that Hawkeye malarkey. Surgery was nowhere near as glamorous as I thought it would be, what with all that fetishistic arm washing that lasted an age. Lathering up your forearms, holding them upright like a priest before the consecration, then the rapid interdigitational rubbing. This was a drag even if it was an imperative. Pulling on a solid metal retractor in someone's abdomen for two hours was hard, boring work.

And the anaesthetists, good bourgeois all, would sit at the top end of the patient reading the *Glasgow Herald*, nodding in agreement with the reactionary rubbish it printed. Every now and then the surgeon would curse, but I was spared the knife-throwing madness that some of my mates encountered. They'd be daydreaming in theatre letting a clamp slip when all of a sudden the boss would flare in anger and go all King of Fling and impale a pillow on a corner seat with a tossed scalpel. The pillow now left scarred, slashed like a canvas by Lucio Fontana.

You need functional parietal lobes to become a surgeon. Your brain needs to be good at telling your hands what to do. Mine isn't. I tie my shoelaces about ten times a day. Every time I'm on a plane after landing I notice my lace undone as I disembark. This seriously pisses off the crowds trying to squeeze past me on thon connecting tube thing as I bend to fix my shoe. If you want to select out medical students appropriate for surgical training then just watch them tying their shoes or putting on a tie. A mere ten seconds of effort that could save an individual years of heartache after they're told, aged thirty-seven, that their career in surgery is over because they can't cut; they can't do knots.

Physicians are doctors who can't cut. Generally speaking. But we get the best stories because we talk to our patients. Surgeons, generally speaking, don't.

At one point on the rotation they sent me to a plastic surgery hospital a few miles outside the city limits, bordering on the countryside. Here you shared the on-call rota with a GP on a one-in-two. On call every second night. Jeez, not again. Nights on were purgatorial; you were alone covering the vast area of the hospital; hikes between the wards across fields. There were no registrars above you; the consultants were all sat at home. I don't think I saw a consultant other than the guy who removed my tumour (Gus McGrouther: a *great* doctor) the whole month I was there. Our job was to write up analgesics and narcotics and to be available if some unfortunate had an arrest. This never happened when I was there: being the one man in a one-man arrest team is no fun. But you would get called at night and this could be very scary. I never knew about skin flaps until I worked there. One night I was called to see a man who had an oral cancer and when I switched on his bedside lamp I nearly jumped up in fright at the sight of this taut piece of skin, this flap, which stretched from his chest wall to his jaw.

My leiomyosarcoma was removed and then reviewed by the histologists. Gus McGrouther told me he wanted to be on the safe side and cut another, wider, ellipse of skin. This he did with real skill and care and I remain in great debt to his intervention. He became a highly esteemed professor who treated many of the victims of the 1999 London nail bomb attacks. Some white supremacist murderer killed three people and injured 140. Gus said: 'The desire of the hospital is to reverse the evil of this act.' My wife and I had a night off in Soho that very evening, in a restaurant nearby, but the first we knew about it was when my dad phoned a couple of hours after it happened to see if we were in town.

When I was a surgical house officer my future wife would come over to the plastics hospital on her days off and in the quiet afternoons we would watch Ceefax together, pages of digital information on the TV screen prior to the internet. Big fun. Having the tumour, being aware of it, had meant that my life felt as if someone had pressed a giant pause button on my existence. That's what doctors need to remember when they talk to patients about cancer: the pause button on life. But now it was press-play time again, I could make plans with her.

And for that I owe another debt to a lady now long gone called Rachel Clemmons. This tired old woman belonged to the small Jewish community that still lived in the Gorbals, an era, a world, described with great tenderness by the writer Ralph Glasser. My own grandmother would sing 'My Yiddishy Mama' to us as children and I often used to wonder if my unknown great-grandmother might possibly have been Jewish. Poor old Rachel had had a stroke and she was bedbound on our medical ward. Dr Hastie told me she needed fed because she couldn't swallow and I was to put a nasogastric tube down her throat. I needed a nurse to help me.

The nurse unpacked the thin tube and handed it over. I leant over Rachel and warned her that this would be a bit uncomfortable and maybe a little bit tickly. The tube went into one of her nostrils and I fed it cleanly down into her stomach. Rachel's pale, tired eyes, clouded with their cataracts, flipped from looking at me on to the nurse and then back to me again. Satisfied I'd got the tube in the right place, I looked up at the nurse. She wore one of those white caps with her blonde hair tied in a ponytail at the back: this time the cap had a thin light blue band that meant she was a student. I thanked her and looked into her eyes for the first time. Blue: as blue as the sea at Troon on a bright summer's day.

I'm thinking now of those popular pulp romance novels about doctors and nurses; it began just like that. Like those ones with the covers that Richard Prince does paintings of, the ones where the couples wear caps and masks. He gives them titles like *Aloha Nurse, Debutant Nurse* or *Doctor's Nurse*. Sonic Youth used one as an album cover. He asked $50k for them when they first appeared in 2003, but they didn't sell back then. One called *Overseas Nurse* sold later this decade for over $8 million. Love stories are popular.

I said no more to her, the blonde-haired girl with cobalt-blue eyes.

A few nights later I saw her again in the canteen; there was no one else there, and she was reading. I managed to get a glimpse of the cover, *Mila 18* by Leon Uris, apparently a decent novel about the Holocaust.

There was something of *Seven Brides for Seven Brothers* amongst my male friends in those first few months after qualifying. We had come down from the desolate highlands of our medical studies in loveless solitude and, rather pathetically, went in search of love. All very Catholic: another far-off world. The impecunious days of living on a grant were now gone; we were salaried. We could ask a girl out.

At university as single men our idea of a night on the town was to hit a dive called the Berlin Bar under Queen Street Station. This was not the Berghain; this was not the KitKatClub. But it was handy for the train home. The Berlin Bar was a pit where we would eke out a couple of pints over two hours. The waitresses wore fishnet stockings: some sexist manager's desperate idea of conjuring up Weimar excess. But now qualified and with money in our pockets we could wine and dine at the likes of the Spaghetti Factory. Flash.

At a staff dance, with the help of an improbable Cupid-like intermediary called Josephine McGarvey, we got talking. Later we had our first night out at the Warren Pizza. A dumb Tolstoy reference – a suitably literary choice, I guessed, for someone reading *Mila 18*. The culinary delights at the Warren Pizza were more in keeping with those Solzhenitsyn might have endured in the Gulag. The Warren Pizza was not like some exquisite banquet featured in *Anna Karenina*. I'm reliably informed that I had not ironed my shirt. I walked her home; she let me kiss her on the cheek. I bounced down the road as weightless as Buzz Aldrin. Like the current number one hit had it – giant steps are what you take. Walking on the moon.

5

NEUROLOGY FOR MEDIEVALISTS

The summer of 1984 I moved up a grade and relocated to the South Side of the city, where there were nine of us acting as senior house officers. We each had a junior house officer below us. We were now bosses ourselves. But there were no registrars above us: this was very unusual. There were three on each team, a JHO, an SHO and a consultant. None of the nine SHOs had passed the MRCP exam fully and so they could not be promoted to the registrar grade. All registrars have to be MRCP: Members of the Royal College of Physicians. Thus there were no juniors with MRCP covering the Southern General's medical wards. And this was a teaching hospital. The responsibility was daunting; we would have to do most, if not all, of the invasive procedures.

But there was one major positive. I'd go from a one-in-two rota, sometimes on call for over 100 hours per week, down to a one-in-nine. *One day on in every nine?* Ya beauty.

The first part of the rotation was with the neurologists. I'd read a few books by Oliver Sacks and was greatly looking forward to working with the really, *really* clever doctors. Even with their bow ties.

A coincidence. I've just read this in *On the Move*, Sacks's autobiography: 'But at fourteen or fifteen, inspired by my school biology teacher and by Steinbeck's *Cannery Row*, I thought I would like to become a marine biologist.' As said, I too fancied being a marine biologist when I hit double figures. That glossy book of marine life off the Great Barrier Reef with all those beautifully coloured photographs: the brain coral with all its sulci; that shot of a half-chewed manta ray. Odd too that it was Steinbeck who was my own introduction to adult reading. I wasn't quite ready yet for my dad's copy of *My Life and Loves* by Frank Harris. As a boy I was tiring of the infinite *Just William* stories and the zoological exploits of Willard Price's Hal and Roger Hunt as they dashed around the planet in rattling yarns like *Diving Adventure*. I remember seeing the spines of the various Steinbeck novels and taking several from the East Kilbride library just after reaching secondary school. The title *The Moon Is Down* fascinated me, but I can't recall what it was about. I was more inspired by *Tortilla Flat* with its cast of wine-guzzling boozed-up chancers.

Underage drinking began for me not long after, when I was thirteen. We would get our hands on a stash: the tallest of my schoolmates, John Duffy, had a bum-fluff moustache and he could get served at an offie. We drank cans of heavy and made for the bosky green hills and a small valley we called 'The Glen'. Here we waded in the shallow waters of the Rotten Calder, a river where we saw heron and woodpeckers. Mildly pished after climbing, we looked out at a necklace of concrete Los Angeles-style roundabouts, those polo mints that circumference our modernist new town. A fat old sun in the sky set over St Leonards.

Sacks also talks of his lack of intellectual self-confidence when he started university: this was easy for me to recognise. I remembered that sinking feeling all too well as I struggled to make sense of something called the Frank-Starling Law. Like Sacks, I found I was doing almost no general reading as a medical student. There was no time. Essentially, we had to cram the names of parts of the body into our heads, *all* of them, and learn how they worked together, and do the lot in just two years. But instinctively you knew that this alone would not be enough to understand 'man'. My head was a mass of anatomical and physiological facts. Where was the organ of Zuckerkandl? What did the pineal gland actually *do*?

Consciously I knew I was a bore. All I could talk about (at any gathering) related to naming: the names of hormones or neurons or blood vessels. Or about how many hours I'd studied the night before. Folks don't want to hear that at parties. Folks don't want to hear about the Bohr effect at a disco. I didn't want to be a Bohr effect bore. I had to read some other stuff again and get a life.

Rescue was at hand. Robert Hughes, a gruff Australian on the TV, would teach me about modern art in his series called *The Shock of the New*. As a young man I loved his no-bullshit precision of expression. He could be fearlessly rude about sacred cows. He said Dalí was no good after he hit thirty-five; that Warhol was rubbish after he got shot. He appeared to hold artists to account. This was pungent criticism, art opinion as spiky as punk rock, or so it seemed to me at the time.

My neurology consultant is called Higgins and is another Irishman. He's garrulous, a braggart and a boor. His registrar Thomas (the neurologists *do* have registrars) is a medievalist trying out a second career in medicine. Thomas trained at Oxford and affects a languid Brideshead air; he has a neatly trimmed beard that makes him look like a prelate. Thomas also points out the finger deficiency in Govan, an inevitable result of poor safety practice in the shipyards.

He is proud to show all ten of his digits by wriggling them around as he makes this observation. Thomas is researching a rare ophthalmic sign, something recherché known as the Holmes-Adie pupil, and freely admits that his studies are of little practical value adding: 'It makes a change from Duns Scotus.'

Thomas makes the regular habit of doing another circuit of the ward immediately after Higgins has finished his own round and had left the ward. Thomas *has* to do this in order to placate upset patients. They need to be talked to again because not a few are fuming.

Higgins's ward rounds are... chaotic, a masterclass in disorder, discord and insensitive communication. I watch aghast as he asks a sixteen-year-old with a recently diagnosed brain tumour what hand he writes with. He gets an answer: 'Left.'

Higgins replies: 'You must be a homosexual.'

Higgins promptly turns and walks on to the next patient. A colleague tells me that on another occasion he intimidated a nervous young nurse on the round and said something that implied she was into oral sex. I've no idea how he gets away with it. I mention this to some seniors in another hospital. They don't either.

Higgins dresses like a dandy, delights in telling me that he buys his pink shirts on Jermyn Street. His accent is Dublin patrician. Another Dubliner who thinks he is an heir to Wilde. I bet the real Buck Mulligan, Oliver St John Gogarty, was like this rude neurologist. Getting away with insults and general cheeky smart-arsery. Higgins is much more of a Mulligan figure than Gerry, my old gastroenterologist mentor, with his benign *You're not a fuckin' comedian* advice.

Thomas the Oxonian is sympathetic when I tell him I've got a lumbar puncture to do on a woman, one of Higgins's patients, who has clear psychosomatic symptomatology. Thomas listens to my moans in silence and nods in sympathy like a priest. He whispers to me: 'Tap the evil spirits from her back, JDQ.'

Higgins is back the next morning and tells me to run an infusion of lignocaine into a man with tinnitus. I'm incredulous. Why should we give a man with some ringing in his ears an anti-dysrhythmic drug I've only ever used at cardiac arrests?

'Lignocaine for tinnitus?'

'Sure, I read about it in *Brain*. Ding-dong.'

Ding-dong? A trial he's read in a neurology journal where the number to treat is given as something ludicrously small as n = three in all likelihood. Higgins is a dabbler. Somehow I manage to talk him out of it.

He develops a habit of grabbing me for endocrine advice: he's worked out that I can glean some sense from these numbers, these blood results, the levels of hormones he gets reports about. He gets reams of these because he has unthinkingly ticked several boxes on a blood request form: 'Jesus, Johnny!'

'What is it?'

'What am I to do with this?'

He shows me a result: a very low white count, a profound case of neutropenia. This is a dangerously low level that could result in overwhelming sepsis. I'm shocked: 'That's worrying.'

'I know! What should I do, *Jesus, JESUS*?'

'Is the patient on anything?'

He looks sheepish. 'Yes.'

'Well, what then?'

'Ah… well, they were feeling pretty tired and I thought they had ME. Maybe there's an autoimmune component. So I thought: *ding-dong*. I'd try to suppress their immune system. I looked in the formulary and I thought I'd try a bit of azathioprine. Was that OK?'

No, it was not OK. ME, myalgic encephalomyelitis, is now more commonly known as chronic fatigue syndrome and it's still an ill-defined and obscure condition with much that remains uncertain about its causes, never mind its management. Azathioprine is generally used for pretty heavy immunosuppression, like preventing rejection in patients who have undergone kidney or heart transplantation. I've no idea why Higgins decided to experiment with this drug. He's panicking now: 'What might happen?'

'Well, they might end up needing a bone marrow transplant.' I'm giving him the worst-case scenario. 'And they could die.'

'Oh, Jesus, Mary and Joseph!'

Somehow, with prayers and divine intervention perhaps, the white count came up.

The start of another week and Higgins is back. The Dubliner is taking the Lord's name in vain again: 'Jesus, what should I do Johnny? I've got this young guy who can't get it up and he's blaming me!'

'What? He's impotent? How come you're seeing him?'

'Well, he came along to the clinic and complained that his muscles were getting a bit bigger and that he was getting a bit hairier and so I thought it must be due to excess testosterone. *Ding-dong.* So I put him on something I looked up in the BNF.'

He means the British National Formulary. He persists in 'looking up' the BNF for his own private amusement, like he's some thirteenth-century alchemist searching for a new spell: the physician as magician. Maybe the surgeons were right about us all along. What has Higgins gone for this time? Then he says this to me: 'I thought, *ding-dong*, his muscles are enlarging because he must be making too much testosterone.'

Too much testosterone? A young guy making *too much* testosterone: what is he *on* about?

Actually, there is a super-rare condition called testotoxicosis caused by a pituitary tumour that overstimulates the testicles. You get bollocks the size of a bull. You look like Buster Gonad from *Viz* magazine. Carrying your knackers around in a wheelbarrow. I've only seen pictures in textbooks: never saw it for real in my entire career. Thankfully testotoxicosis is outlandishly uncommon. Generally you don't need a wheelbarrow.

Higgins is a neurologist, not an endocrinologist. Again I'm aghast. Again I'm worried what he might have used, but I ask him first: 'How old is this guy?'

'Twenty-two.'

'*Twenty-two!*'

I've frightened him with my obvious incredulity. And then I hazard a guess as to what he might have tried out on the young lad: 'You've not given him cyproterone, surely?'

'Yes, that's the one. Was that not an OK thing to do?'

'Well, if you want to chemically castrate someone, then yes.'

'*Castration?* Oh, Mother of Mary what have I done?'

I'm tempted to say he's dinged the guy's dong. Luckily for him the testosterone recovers once the lad comes off the cyproterone. Presumably his erectile function improves too, because we hear no more of it from Higgins.

Another day on the neurology ward with Higgins doing the round: his confidence has returned and he bounces back as chirpy as a terrier puppy. He's just as irritating. That bullying tendency of his comes out once again and he mocks his registrar, ignores the rest of us. He's enjoying the humiliation of Peterson, a bright lad with a nervous stutter. Higgins, secure in his delusions, thinks he is educating him. He asks mock-seriously: 'What's the best bedside test for neurological functionality?'

Peterson stumbles: 'I'm n-not sure, Dr Higgins.'

Peterson is meek. He twiddles his own spotted bow tie, the clue he wants to become a consultant neurologist in time. Higgins raises his voice: 'Get them to hop! C'mon, Peterson, get hopping! Hop, man, hop!'

And poor Peterson hops on one leg right there in the corridor; the nurses are giggling now. It's someone else's turn to be bullied.

I never felt comfortable around the patients on the neurology ward with the condition myasthenia gravis: MG. Like SLE, this disease seemed to be dangerously unpredictable but predictable to the extent that the patients liked to go off when I was on call. They were either on too large or too small a dose of the drugs that could improve the disease. In both cases respiratory arrest could happen: sudden termination of breathing. In effect this was Ondine's curse. Ondine's curse for real.

Then there was panic and an arrest call. Sudden squeezing of that horrid black rubber bag. Sudden bagging. Sudden decisions on dosages of obscure drugs. What did T. S. Eliot say about showing you fear in a handful of dust? No, I'll show you real fear: real fear is covering a ward full of myaesthenics.

Neurologists couldn't seem to cure a thing and as I can't stop myself from saying again, they persistently wore bow ties. But thank God for Oliver Sacks: he was my real neurology teacher.

For years and years, I would teach students about how some stroke patients would have a deficiency in their field of vision, one that meant they would ignore half of the food on their plates. A tale pinched straight from Sacks, of course. Patter theft. And I'd dwell too on the existential significance Sacks taught me about these deficiencies: how an additional chunk of the world had just disappeared for these poor people. I'd ask the students: what was going on behind them right now? What was out of range of their visual field? Then I'd ask how could they be sure, be certain, that there was not a man with a gun out of sight, out of mind? Now imagine that this blank space, this dead zone we can confront only by turning our heads, imagine that this dead zone was now enlarged, that the whole world had been made smaller, by this visual field defect, by this (lovely term) *homonymous hemianopia.* These strangely beautiful labels. It was not just science that attracted me to medicine; it was words too: *phaeochromocytoma, acromegaly, sartorius, cremaster.*

Daily more words that obscurely sang out, words that held secret knowledge. Despite what Sacks had taught me in his case histories, his enthusiasm for the minutiae of brain pathology, I could not share the frank indifference some neurologists had for their caseload of incurables. I decided, reluctantly, against a career in neurology.

6

HARTY

I went from neurology to elderly care: from a gleaming '70s Le Corbusier tower block to some Nissen huts. Elderly care was very much a Cinderella specialty in those days. One consultant I worked for, an elderly lady herself and near retirement, tut-tutted at an old fella in a bed, another former shipyard worker, who had what she called 'the dropsy'. She lectured us about William Withering and his first trials using digitalis: it all felt a bit eighteenth century working with her; maybe she had known Withering.

Her accent was posh Kelvinside and, daydreaming, I'd imagine her offering me a nub of snuff while we inspected the elephantine legs of the old fitter. She turned to me and ordered: 'Get me a syringe, some local... and a bucket.'

A bucket? I'd heard right. With some effort we raised the man's heavy bloated legs, propped his feet on a chair and placed the bucket underneath the bridge his limbs made. She then swiftly jabbed here and there with the anaesthetic into his weighty, waterlogged calves. We waited a few minutes. She magicked a scalpel and some other implements and then made several quick slashes on the tensed skin of the man's calves. She watched patiently as pink thinned blood and water dripped into the bucket below. Her chin raised to the sky as she announced proudly: 'Now that's how you treat heart failure.'

I think she used something called Southey's tubes: fine-calibre plastic cannulae that she stuck under the skin like a picador. Horrific.

I've just googled Southey: Reginald Southey (1835–99). A Bart's man and a lifelong friend of the Reverend Charles L. Dodgson aka Lewis Carroll. Southey, it says here, encouraged dodgy Dodgson to take up photography. *Encouraged.* I'm guessing Southey didn't highlight that fact on his CV.

Thank God for modern pharmacology. No buckets needed now. And then after my spell with the knife-wielding matadora it was back to covering the general medical wards.

Being on call overnight was challenging when there was no medical registrar. If it was just you and one house officer, any practical procedures that needing doing – well, they were firmly in your domain even if there were up to ten people still waiting to be seen in A+E. With only two consultant cardiologists (on a one-in-two rota, of course) we were reluctant to call on them at four in the morning if, say, someone needed a pacemaker inserted. A 'temporary wire' was the term we used. We'd give it a go. *Put a wire in them.*

See one, do one, teach one. That was the training mantra that we grew up with. *Here's how you do an appendicectomy, JDQ. Watch and learn. Tomorrow night you can do one yourself.*

One of the cardiologists was jokingly known as Harty. Apparently he had once eaten some heart as a gag. Ox heart, I assume; the alternative is too outrageous to contemplate. Harty was more approachable than his taciturn colleague. Harty was a genial soul who loved Bach and would have tapes of recordings by Neville Marriner scattered over the back seats of his car. He smoked a pipe and thought nothing of taking this out his pocket during ward rounds and playing with it obsessively, even when unlit. Then he would take out his pocketknife to remove bits of baccy gubbins that had lodged under his nails. He'd do that at that end of the bed while talking to patients. You could do that sort of thing before MRSA, before *C. dif* (*Clostridium difficile*), before Covid-19. His manner was calm and deliberate and, aside from the baccy shenanigans, he impressed me greatly.

One afternoon a man in his early twenties came into A+E with palpitations. We hooked him up to a monitor and did an ECG. He was (in the deliberately understated words we habitually used) *rattling along*. His heart rate was over 150 bpm. I gave him the standard treatment of the time, a drug called verapamil, and… nothing happened. He was still rattling along.

I can't remember much else about that young man now. Was he tall or short, was he fat or thin? He can't have been fat: this I would recall because it would have made the procedure even tougher. He was an otherwise fit young man, of that I'm sure. Black hair? Who knows. Job or unemployed? Job, I think. Wife? Maybe. Kids? Maybe not. *Rattling along*. Rate now 180, blood pressure just about holding. But I do remember thinking: *This is not good*. I needed Harty.

There he was idling down one of the interminably long corridors of the hospital, pipe switching from hand to mouth for a quick chew. I told him the story succinctly. He listened carefully, heard about the verapamil, paused, took his pipe from his lips and pointed the stem at me and said: 'Fast atrial pace him.'

He said bye, turned and walked away.

The phrase buzzed in my head: *fast atrial pace him*. And with it the image of the young man. Shit! He wasn't a man, he was a boy really. Fast atrial pace: what did that even mean? And by the time my brain began screaming – *Hey, wait a minute!* – Harty had gone.

I ran up to the coronary care unit where the lad had been transferred and told the nurses what the boss had suggested. The sister in charge, ahem, took charge: 'Done one before?'

'What, fast atrial pacing?'

'Aye.'

'Naw.'

'It's nae bother. We'll talk and walk you through it.'

And this they did.

I can't recall explaining the procedure to the young guy: hell, I hardly knew what it involved myself. I put some local anaesthetic into the hollow of his elbow and, once he couldn't feel me jabbing him, cut down through the skin and fat to find the blue hue of the brachial vein. I was scared witless about the brachial artery bounding away right next door. *Rattling along.* I found the vein.

I had gowned up of course, gloved and masked. And underneath all that I had to don a lead apron. The phrase 'a lead weight' is apt. This was like working with a two-year-old kid hanging onto your back. The sister, a trouper if ever there was one, my new mum, a smarter mum that I needed right here, right now, handed me the wire. I made an incision in the vein and through the opening threaded the wire upwards to the lad's neck. *Put a wire in them.* Here we paused and other members of the team moved the mobile screening device into position. This was a heavyweight machine that could image the heart by X-ray and the wire I was attempting to steer into one of the chambers (the atrium), hence atrial pacing. The fast bit remained a mystery to me.

At my foot was a pedal I could press on to get an image from the TV screen above our heads. I was to restrict the time imaging given the exposure risk of radiation. OK. Now I could see that we were just below the lad's clavicle. The wire was moving upwards with pleasing ease. Although I remain haunless, I can understand the pleasure that many get from manual dexterity; I wish I had it. My foot hit the pedal to switch on the screen again: the wire had turned southwards and was beginning to flick in rhythm with the heart. The wire looked to be flicking as fast as hummingbird wings. Power off, I turned to Sister and asked: 'Are we in?'

'I think so.'

'I'll screen again.'

We looked at the image together, the whipping motion of the wire curled up against the wall of the atrium. Sister looks at me. Her eyes are all I can see of her face given that she is masked up too; she winks and says: 'We're in.'

What happens next is that one of the other nurses assisting connects my end of the wire to a box. A black box that I have seen the cardiologists playing around with; I've seen them use it at cardiac arrests before. Cardiologists like to affect a sub-zero cool. When I watched them handling pacing boxes at arrests, I was reminded of poker players in Hollywood movies; Paul Newman types with a steady hand. And they would always be laconic. They'd talk in one-word sentences. *Capture. Pacing.*

I could never be a cardiologist.

The box has switches, knobs and dials. Black dials like the ones I'd seen Eno twiddling on *Top of the Pops*. One of these can be turned to speed up the heart rate. This is why we use pacing wires in elderly patients with complete heart block, where the heart rate is down as low as 30 bpm. Our lad is still rattling around 180.

Now here comes the really fast bit, the fast atrial pacing bit. I'm inside the guy's heart with the wire. And now I'm sure we're in I nod to the nurse with the box. She turns one of the knobs that stimulates the wire to pace the heart at a speed *above* the current rate our lad is tolerating. The idea then is to override the actual atrial pacemaker deep in the muscle, the myocardium, of our lad's heart, and then, *click*, turn the pacing box switch off again in the hope, the sincere hope, the screaming out to God above hope, that the heart rate of this poor young man will return to normal.

Immediately something's wrong. Sister has seen the ECG monitor change. The shape of the beats, the complexes of electrical activity, has been narrow, as with my working diagnosis: a supraventricular tachycardia (SVT). These complexes are now very wide: this is now a ventricular tachycardia (VT).

Two initials you never want to hear. VT. You don't want to hear that. Here are two more: VF. Ventricular fibrillation. These are pre-terminal events. You do not want to be the cause of VT or VF in a young person.

VT. *FUCK!!!* Inside my head is yelling *fuckfuckfuck*: pull back, pull back, get that fucking wire back into the atrium.

'Switch off.'

Sister is calm. Her colleague turns the knob back, the trace narrows, the lad is back into an SVT. I pull the wire back, reimage, try again and this time it works. He's reverted into sinus rhythm: 60 bpm. Phew.

My own heart rate is over 100, I'm depleted of adrenaline: it's as if someone has squeezed my adrenal glands, as if some invisible hand has reached into my belly and squashed them. At the same time that toddler is still sat on my back, the weight of the apron now wearily pressing down on me like a sack of coal.

Years later a better drug than verapamil came along, one that reduced the need for fast atrial pacing by some margin. *See one, do one, teach one.* Yeah, right. Cool.

The tyranny of cool: the cardiologists were *soooo* cool. The senior house officer, Spike (so named because of his post-punk hairdo), dined at the Malmaison. Spike knew when the Pomerol was corked and wasn't afraid to tell the sommelier. The senior registrar, Adam, looked like Sting, the ace-face version of Sting from *Quadrophenia*. Another registrar, Alan, wore a red T-shirt at Christmas with a white slogan that read H. F. H. *Ho fuckin ho*. Yet another registrar, Simpo, was a big Rangers fan and had a drawl like Sean Connery's. He'd sometimes impersonate Sean. He'd be derogatory about buying a season ticket for Celtic Park: *shelling your shoal to the shlime of humanity*.

All the cardiologists spoke very deliberately, slowly: they all drawled. That drawl they had: I wanted it too. I wanted to drawl like a cardiologist. Why not copy them and cultivate a groovy drawl like Simpo's or maybe Davy Henderson's, say? Davy, the singer from the Fire Engines and Win: a drawl like Davy's conveyed seriousness of purpose, depth, hard-won wisdom, cool. I imagined the cardiologists as our beat poets with their Burroughs monotones, facing death with dark irony, equanimity. You can hear a cardiologist's mind drawling as they face death: *death, that old faker*.

Cardiologists knew when to act: cardiologists loved Lee Marvin and Chic Murray. Chic was their idea of a comedian. Deadpan one-liners. They were laconic, hard to get. They believed in the tyranny of cool.

I could never have been a cardiologist.

I thought that trying to appear cool was uncool. Cool was being indifferent to being cool. I thought I was cooler than them. Which was *really* uncool.

But they taught me the mysteries of the ECG. The electrical patterns of the heart as seen on a paper tracing: the heart going for a walk with a line. Sometimes the walk was more like a sprint, as with the tachycardias; sometimes a dawdle like the bradycardias. Knowing how to decode an ECG was a kind of occult knowledge. ECGs: you got the deep sense that they went to the heart of things. Other juniors badgered you to help interpret them. Understanding ECGs was *sehr* cool: U waves, bundle branch block, axis deviation, VT, AF, VF.

Cardiology was an overwhelmingly male specialty in the '80s, now being belatedly corrected this century.

August 1985 and I'm about to start my second year as SHO. I have exams to pass if I want to pursue my wish to become a consultant. 1 August is when the new doctors start, the new JHOs, the house-dogs. On 2 August at seven in the morning I'm in bed at home. I'm not on call, but the phone rings and I hear the voice of one of my SHO colleagues. She's crying. She stammers out: 'I don't know what to do with this guy.'

'Hang on a sec. Say again. Is it a patient?'

'No. It's one of the new doctors, that guy Jim.'

'Who?'

'You know him. Jim! Jim: the big guy, the army guy. He's completely mad... he's running around the place screaming his head off.'

She's telling me this early because I'm on call with Jim that day, 2 August 1985: the worst day of my career.

I meet Jim after I've finished another consultant-less ward round; he's late. And he *is* big. Jim is big and broad; he looks like he does a lot of exercise. He's wearing a camouflage jacket instead of a white coat. And he's talking about guns. Guns, not patients; he seems unconcerned about patients. What he cares about is... weaponry.

Guns. Revolvers and rifles. Different makes. I'm reminded of the sleazy salesman in *Taxi Driver* going on about a .44 Magnum. *It's a real monster. It'll stop a car at a hundred yards.* I ask Jim if he has seen anyone yet in A+E and he says yes and so I ask him to tell me about the patient: has he clerked him or her in yet? Has he written anything down? He nods and shows me a piece of paper with some squiggles on it. This looks like abstract art; this makes the scrawls of Cy Twombly look a model of lucidity. I redden: those sorely tried adrenal glands of mine are being wrung out again; they're giving off another squeeze of adrenaline.

Before I can say anything else the arrest page screams into life, EEEE-EEEE-EEEE, and then Jim starts screaming too. Yelling like a banshee. He's now running this way and that like some cartoon dervish, like that animated Tasmanian devil. A voice emerges from the page: *Testing, testing, switchboard testing.* I tell him to calm down, to relax, that we are not needed, not now. He takes deep breaths and eventually he seems more at ease.

And then asks me this: 'What's your favourite shotgun?'

I tell him honestly that I have little knowledge of guns. He explains that he is in the Territorial Army and hence his camo jacket. I say to him maybe it would be better if he changed into a white coat because although the ward might look like the front line of a war zone it's not an *actual* battle scene. I also suggest that I carry his page and he smiles and says, yes, that might be a good idea.

I sneak away and phone switchboard. I'm firm, rushed: 'Do me a real favour. On no account contact this guy Jim and ask him to do *anything*, OK?'

As ever, switch are great and don't bug Jim. And then I head in search of Harty. Who hears me out in his office when I find him. He sits forward and listens carefully, all the while the unlit pipe clamped in his mouth. The camo jacket, the guns, the screaming, the illegible scribbling. I'm succinct in my diagnosis. I know very little about psychiatry and madness but I'm as sure as I've ever been about any-thing in this life that our young man Jim is acutely psychotic. And he's wearing a doctor's badge. Harty looks up, he's gruff; he wants to be reasonable: 'It's only his first day, JDQ. Give him a chance.'

Maybe I'm exaggerating. Harty is right to be cautious. I walk down another one of those long corridors slowly, dejected, close to despair. How can I do my job *and* Jim's job? How can I work with Travis Fucking Bickle? And then the fast page trills into life yet again. EEEE-EEEE-EEEE. Not a test this time: the action really is in A+E. A middle-aged man has ruptured his aorta. He needs life-saving surgery but now he has arrested.

We try. We fail. And then I'm told that he is the father of one of my colleagues, another SHO. I have to tell him that his dad has just died.

Walking back to the medical wards after this disaster, I meet Jim. More crazy shit about what a certain type of bullet can do. I'm more convinced now that I need to sort him out. I need help, I cannot have Jim on my back for another eighteen hours, have him running around yelling nonsense overnight. With the utmost reluctance I decide to go over the head of my consultant, to bypass Harty, and call in a psychiatrist.

Thankfully the psychiatrist is extremely helpful. He asks me to bring Jim to a room and, amazingly (when I eventually find him), he agrees to come along. The patients meanwhile are piling up at A+E. A manager phones to say we are low in beds. I take a deep breath in. The psychiatrist calls me about an hour later and tells me that he is admitting Jim. He thinks he might be acutely schizophrenic.

I need someone else to be on call with me tonight (I can't do it on my own), so I have to go to the mess and press-gang a junior. One quickly agrees: the camaraderie of medicine is often inspirational.

And then I'm crossing a car park just after 5 p.m. and spot Kris, now a senior registrar, leaving. He winds his window down and I tell him about my day. He smiles and says: 'Character building, JDQ, *character building.*'

Kris tells me the next day that about a week before starting their first jobs all the new JHOs were addressed by the Dean. At the end of his talk about what they should expect as new doctors, the Dean asked if anyone had any questions. Jim, Territorial Army recruit and gun nut, put his hand up and asked: *What do we do for bins?*

I was told everyone in the room laughed. All 200 who had taken courses on psychiatry. All were about to look after the sick in a week's time but none of them could see what was going on in front of their faces. And what about the Dean? He didn't see it either. I too would learn the hard way. Real trouble can be staring you in the face and you can be completely blind to it.

A year later I moved back to the Royal as a registrar, having been successful in the MRCP exam. Kris had rotated back too as a senior registrar. One morning he tells me the terrible news: 'Jim returned to work two weeks ago. They said he was OK. But apparently he was going on about guns again and talking about shooting a consultant. Yeah, taking one of us out! Yesterday the cleaners couldn't get into his room.'

'Oh no...'

'They knocked and knocked and eventually got security to break the door down. He'd shot himself.'

Two years after I heard this Jim came back into my mind because he bore a striking physical resemblance to Michael Ryan, that crazed mass murderer in Hungerford who shot dead sixteen people before turning the gun on himself. There was the same hunter's beanie hat that I'd seen Jim pop into his pocket, the same naff camo jacket, the same blank stare, the same scrawny, ill-kempt beard.

Talking about shooting a consultant.

Decades later I'd go on and work for the Deanery *because* of this experience. The Deanery is in charge of trainee welfare. I did not want a repetition. We must try to prevent these tragedies from happening again.

We married, honeymooned on Malta listening to Colourbox and Scritti Politti, came home and got a small flat wedged between a railway line and a canal. We made a train trip to West Berlin in the winter of 1986 and froze in our thin cagoules as we trekked up an empty Unter den Linden towards a deadened Alexanderplatz. There were very few shops and there was nothing worth eating. We had to spend our DDR marks before heading back across Checkpoint Charlie and so ordered double Blue Lagoons in some dive. I remembered a building that had a sign above it that read Ost. We were in the East behind the Iron Curtain and it felt cold and scary.

We were being watched. If one of these people, a Stasi person, say, had told me that much of my 21st-century future would be based here I would have panicked: I would have assumed that the Russians had won the Cold War. That's how daft we were back then.

When I got home to Glasgow I'd trudge back and forth in the driving rain. I'd go to work by train listening to Bowie's *Low* on my Sony Walkman. I had not yet learned to drive. My driving test would be the last exam I'd ever sit.

On the South Side of the city I worked with Jock, a kippered old wizard of a consultant physician who chain-smoked and sat cross-legged, his heron-thin legs draped with polyester trousers stained by fag ash that he'd occasionally brush aside. Jock was internationally respected, knew everything there was to know about vitamin B12, and I learned loads from observing his calm, unruffled manner. He'd seen it all. Jock's younger consultant colleague would go on to become a PRCP, a president of the RCP. This colleague of Jock's was a small man called McGee who was another of those who wore his white coat tightly buttoned to his neck. Quite a few of the consultants sported that look back then: I'm not sure why. And right enough they did look like a babble of barbers.

McGee was badly myopic and wore bottle-glassed lenses that made him look like a mad scientist, not unlike that guy who runs the Tyrell Corporation in *Blade Runner*. As befits a PRCP he was a terrific clinician. But maybe he knew this all too well and, perhaps unsurprisingly, his intermittent smugness irritated the other colleague on the team, droning Douglas Anderson of the aforementioned rota spat. I remember McGee one day on a round taking a brief look at a patient with a pillar-box red tongue. He turned to me and said quietly: 'Scarlet fever. What… you've never seen that before?'

I don't think I impressed McGee. He always seemed to address me in a manner akin to a bored parent tiring of his charge. I watched him have another on-call argument with his whiny colleague Douglas; it was clear the future president would have his way.

McGee was incredulous when I told him I thought about dying every day: '*Every day*? How old are you?'

'Twenty-five.'

'*Twenty-five*? I'm fifty-five and I never think about death. *Never.*'

And with that he went off to talk with another group of dying people on the wards. Death, for him as for Duchamp, was something that only happened to *les autres*.

Spring 1986: I pass my exams and become a member of the Royal College of Physicians. My parents miss the graduation ceremony. I can't recall exactly why – probably something to do with money. By that time they were back from Malta. The money had gone on nights out eating baked timpana pasta. Now they were 500 miles away in Essex, temporarily stuck in Jaywick, of all places. Fucking Jaywick. Have you been there? Jaywick is like a Uruguayan border town that's seen better days. Give it a miss.

The patter theft klaxon has just gone off. Didn't Paul Theroux visit Jaywick on his round-Britain trip, *The Kingdom by the Sea*? I check my copy. He did indeed and said that Jaywick was '...awfully battered, like a seaside slum in Argentina or Mexico. It had the same grubby geniality, the same broken fences.'

Anyway, my folks were temporarily skint. That was their excuse for not heading north for the graduation, I think. Either that or it was the fact that I was now a grown-up married man who didn't need his halo polished any more. They were right not to come. They needed to concentrate on getting out of Jaywick.

I take my wife and Mary, my paternal grandmother, the latter because she kindly let me stay with her as a student. She had been left a house with three bedrooms after her husband, the Tory bantam, died. Mary had always held doctors in ludicrously high esteem, largely because she worked for a surgeon in the 1930s when she was 'in service'. In service was a posh way of saying you were a servant: a cleaner/cook/skivvy/home help. She read the *Express* and would ask me why Hollywood stars always seemed to get cancer. Mary had airs and loved the attention and age-related respect she got from the likes of McGee the PRCP, Gerry, Prof. Fraser and all the other elder physicians in their shiny gowns at the graduation.

With my new title, I secure a job as a registrar. I cross the river again, back to my alma mater, and work with Kris and JBF and Dr Hastie, who is now relieved after the *actual* death of Mrs Bond. As Kris is a senior registrar I can still call him by his first name, but what about the consultants? No, no way: as was the manner in this country at the time, this was the class system in miniature. The real bosses get called 'Doctor' and then their surname. Or you can use their initials if you have been accorded due respect, those three initials. You can call them by their first name only when *you* become a consultant.

I am now a registrar training in diabetes and endocrinology but still have a large general medical inpatient load and remain on call overnight every eight days or so. The registrar controls the show. The medical registrar job is probably the toughest job in the hospital and today in the twenty-first century it is even harder. Applications are down: the young trainees today know how difficult being on at night is for the medical registrar. You are *it*. By that I mean you are in charge of the 'take': you have to coordinate the medical admissions (basically all those cases that do not require the knife, a paediatrician or an obstetrician) and ensure everyone is seen, make sure they have a bed, make sure the diagnosis and plan are correct. Basically you have to do your best to keep all the punters alive until the morning round. That and running to arrests, resuscitating the shocked and getting people transferred to ITU.

The buck, on the ground, stops with you. You *can* phone a friend, you can phone a consultant but... you try not to. You are run ragged. It is a physical job; you pound down those long corridors like Lee Marvin in *Point Blank*. Like Lee, you have to face down any unhelpful colleagues, the clock-watchers, the timewasters, the lazy, and there *are* a few of those. You have to deal with the drunks, the eccied, the psychotics. The noise in A+E is often at a level that is not conducive to thinking clearly, for calculations, for working out doses, say. Pages are going off everywhere, ambulance people are shouting, the drugged party people are yelling, phones are trilling, and then someone will sidle up to you and ask: 'Could you just have a quick look at the patient in room four?'

But there is a buzz. You are in demand; you are in control. It's a young person's game.

JBF calls me, asks me to come to his office for a chat. He is respected but he intimidates some of the more callow juniors because he insists that they tell him the truth about patients, about situations, not what they *think* he wants to hear. He is a stickler for correct spelling (his test of choice being amitriptyline: *three 'i's, JDQ, three 'i's*) and insists that the drug kardex, the list of medications a patient is on, be legible and up to date. He is a clinical pharmacologist who specialises in the side effects of drugs. In time he will chair the national committee on the review of medicines. He is an enemy of spin. I know he is high up in the Edinburgh College. I knock on his door with trepidation. Maybe I've spelt amitriptyline wrong again.

He's affable and offers me a coffee: I'm going to be fired; I know it. Medicine is about fear. John Cale may have sung 'Fear is a man's best friend', but you can have enough of fear. John Cale never worked at the Royal.

Fear of certain clinical situations is very sensible. At night on call I'd lie in bed (if I got there) and, before trying to sleep for an hour or whatever, I'd mentally go through my superstitious routine, imagining all the wards in my head as if counting sheep. And so I'd think about being called to A+E to see someone with a pneumothorax, say. (Numerous books have highlighted that doctors should not, should never, refer to patients as 'the pneumothorax in bed seven' and I agree with this, but when imagining cases that haven't arrived yet they don't have a name, and so it is not unreasonable to think about what you might do if 'a pneumothorax' comes in.) These spirals of demented forecasting, this attempt to outwit fear, to match the controlled pity one has when dealing with a patient with a controlled fear: that was my psychology. If you think the worst is about to happen then it will not happen. Magical thinking. And then weirdly it actually *does* happen. That pregnant woman on the obstetric ward, you forgot about her in your mental checklist, didn't you? So at four in the morning she is the one you will be called to.

The mind wrestling through the night in those dingy on-call rooms and then, miraculously, the dawn light through the threadbare curtain wakes you: you have survived yet another night.

So when JBF gets his secretary to bring us a coffee I'm thinking: He's going to tell me I'm fired. What did I do wrong? That's the unspoken mantra in medicine. *What have I done wrong?*

He sits and removes his glasses, polishes them with a piece of cloth, and I'm struck by his face, now unreadable, its authority now rendered mute. His glasses are such a part of his image that I don't recognise the face I'm now peering at. He looks human again: he even looks... kind. I realise now that this is what people must think when I take off my specs: they don't know what they are seeing. *Oh, that's what he actually looks like.* A stranger.

'So, you are thinking of a career in diabetes and the hormones then?'

I'm secure: I'm not to be fired. This is a career chat. I'm twenty-five and this man will now map out my future.

JBF is chair of the senior registrar committee. Back then getting an SR job (average age around thirty-five) was a virtual guarantee of getting a consultant post in time. Many registrars, on the other hand, didn't progress and had to change careers: some became GPs or left the front line for the pharmaceutical industry. This pattern would change only *after* I became a consultant. The SR grade would be scrapped: the wastage of registrars would be corrected. Nowadays a registrar post (average age around twenty-seven) is, effectively, to be anointed a future consultant. In short, most registrars this century attain career security much earlier. We had severe bouts of career insecurity well into our fourth decades.

JBF knows the future, he knows *my* future; he knows the numbers game. He understands the demographic: how many consultants are about to retire and when they plan to do so. This determines the number of SR posts that will then be advertised. As planner, he knows in what order this will be, because there is a strict rotation of advertised posts between the specialties. In Scotland at that time SR vacancies were not filled on a needs basis as such: appointments were made to whichever specialty happened to be next in line. So if a consultant somewhere in the city retired and an SR got his or her post, the next SR job to be advertised in the city might be in another specialty entirely, cardiology say, because it's their turn.

'You know KOJ just got appointed SR?'

Kay–oh–jay? He means Kris.

'And you know that that means the next diabetes and endocrine SR will not be advertised for some time. Remember Moira is ahead of you by a couple of years.'

Moira was a rarity back then, a woman registrar making a career, quite brilliantly, as a physician. More decades would have to pass before women had anything like a fairer deal in the medical workplace. There's still much work to be done, especially on pay.

I nod.

'So this means that if you want an SR post here in Glasgow you may have to wait. Wait quite a while, I'm afraid.'

Even for a small country, Scotland has only a small number of diabetes consultants. For decades we have been exporters of doctors. I can see in his face that JBF is not enjoying what he has to tell me. I think I can guess his politics and suspect that he might want independence, or at least devolution, for Scotland. This at a time when to hold such views was a minority opinion. I recognise his love for our country, his inner sense that we should stop being dependent. I can see that it pains him to suggest that I may need to become an exile: 'We will back you; we will train you. But you might need to head down south to England for a consultant job. How does that sound?'

Down south. Southbound. I tell him my parents live in Essex but say nothing about Jaywick. And then I lie: 'I've got no problem with that.'

But I have because my wife and her family live in Glasgow and although my family has left for the flatlands of Essex with its easy money, its fascination with gangsters, I have stayed north throughout my university years and my three years as a doctor. This is my city, my country. I don't want to leave.

He smiles, puts his glasses back on. He's JBF again. I've said what I think he wants to hear. Exactly what I've noted others cowed into doing, I've said what he specifically *doesn't* want to hear: a lie. I do have a problem with leaving. But such acceptance is common in medicine. We have to go where the jobs are. Workforce planning is an oxymoron. His advice would be proven right. In time I would leave Scotland.

The months on the wards add up and I'm more confident on the rounds now with JBF: he is a natural contrarian and challenges many of the scuffed pearls of received medical wisdom. *What's your evidence for saying that?* Like a boxer sparring with a weaker opponent, he goads me and I take some hits but then slowly, steadily, I begin to raise my game and catch him the odd, well-timed blow. *You think this is a case of pseudo-hypoparathyroidism, do you?* I realise that he is toughening me up: he knows that I will face opponents in the future who will have none of his gentlemanly restraint, who will play rough: the occasional psychopathic surgeon, the lying sociopaths. I will learn the hard way, as most medics do, that trying to deal with the personality disordered is a tiring, fifteen-round business. JBF teaches me how to pick my fights. Don't go for ones you will lose.

Years later there will be much press about whistleblowing in the NHS. Holding people to account has never been easy. Whistleblowers emerge punch-drunk or ruined. They have splinters of glass removed from their scalps after crashing into invisible ceilings. The odds are stacked against them.

JBF launches my first attempt at research. I'm quick to realise that I'm too indolent and too impatiently skittish to become a real academic. I have been in bars at 2 a.m. listening to professors talk about new binding proteins and know that I lack their scary focus. Academics have the courage to be single-minded. This demands a monk- or nun-like vocation, real dedication. They hide away in their libraries and labs and talk to a handful of people globally, the few that really understand them. Some have no small talk whatsoever. But medicine can only go forward with their selfless efforts. Look in awe at their striving for cures, for vaccines. They blank out the outside world so that *you* might live more safely. At retiral parties often they are the ones who regret not spending enough time with their families.

I collect some data and then JBF asks if I can present the results: in Switzerland!

7

PIKE AT THE BEAU-RIVAGE, OUCHY

'm twenty-six and off with my slides to Lausanne. Slides, those small plastic squares that damage, that crack, so easily; you carry them around in blue boxes. Computers can't come fast enough. I've met the company representatives at the airport. Ah, yes: the company. A pharmaceutical giant is sponsoring the trip. But that's OK because I'm presenting some scientific data, not on a skiing jaunt. It's kosher.

We land and I'm told we have a cab taking us to Ouchy on Lake Geneva. Light rain is drizzling from the grey skies: the lake is still and looks metallic, like molten lead. I pull on a blue cagoule, look down and see that my shoes are scuffed; I need a new pair. I'm wearing an M&S jacket, the tailoring of choice for young registrars. We get out the cab and walk on a recently raked gravel path towards… a palace.

The building is a neo-baroque extravaganza with 168 rooms, conference, banquet and spa facilities. A doorman insists on helping me with my ultra-light bag. I follow him to the lift. We pass floral displays of shocking exuberance. Very wealthy people drift into the reception and my face now burns with shame. I'm acutely aware that scuffed shoes and cagoules and M&S suits are inappropriate here. I'm conscious that everyone staying at the Beau-Rivage has vast wealth and that I am not one of them. I'm on the receiving end of snobbish staring. I do not have any small change for tipping, only bank notes that I'm going to need for a coffee here, and the baggage handler is now hanging around, delaying his exit from my room; another minor humiliation.

Up in my suite I eat a peach nabbed from the overflowing crystal fruit bowl on the table. There's enough fruit here for a family of four: some bananas, three figs, an apple, an orange, and those hairy green things I've never eaten before. From New Zealand, I think. The room has tall windows, beautifully draped; an enormous bed; a God-given view of the lake. A passenger boat chugs past trailing its white wake; there are mountains in the distance. This is some kind of paradise and I should not be here. I tell myself that I have been invited to do my talk, to go through my slides, but I know that I have not earned this degree of privilege. Not really.

The British company representative meets me. He says with some smugness that he gave up being a registrar two years ago: he'd 'had enough of the riff-raff'. Not yet thirty, he has a degree of facial bloating. He expresses himself in a contrived patrician drawl. His affected bearing reminds me of Jeremy Irons starring in the TV version of *Brideshead Revisited*. He had worked as a doctor in London: 'All that madness in A+E, the drunks and the addicts: I just couldn't stand it any longer. So I left and joined the company. Wonderful life. And much better pay, of course. Fancy some pike for lunch? They do it so well here. Pike and a lovely Meursault.'

I'm thinking like a teenager: *What a sell-out!* Sell-out, the ultimate insult if you belonged to the blank generation, *my* generation. I'm a daft sixteen-year-old punk again. Sell-out: I had a picture of

The Clash in my head, Joe Strummer posing with a Brigate Rosse T-shirt in Belfast, the Belfast of the late 1970s, a place of car bombs and kneecappings. Dickhead. Joe Strummer, son of a diplomat, the rock 'n' roll rebel who sang about his daddy being a bank-robber who loved to steal your money. I wondered: how many people currently staying at the Beau-Rivage love to steal your money? Then Joe signed up with CBS Records, CBS! *Sell-outs!*

This drug company pike guy had taken the thirty pieces of silver. Long-dormant Catholic guilt assailed me as I walked around Lausanne, an upright, uptight, Calvinist city. I watch another steamer chug along the lake and hear it toot-tooting: the flag at the stern flutters, a simple white cross on a red background.

From the guide to the hotel: *With a wine list of over 3,000 wines and 75,000 bottles carefully stored and aged.*

And then the menu: *Wild abalone from Brittany.*

What in hell was abalone?

I pass on a trip to the spa and do my talk, a minor study of very little significance, in a room that will, in time, host the negotiations on the US/Iranian nuclear deal. Lunch costs more than I'd spend on food in a month back in Britain. The small embarrassments of the day become increasingly excruciating. There is an air of complicity, of dissipation, of shenanigans. The whole trip is pretty ludicrous.

Back home in Glasgow the steelworks were laying men off in the thousands. The city was being filleted as surely as a Dover sole at the Beau-Rivage. At the same time down in Essex my sister had escaped Jaywick. She now lived in a converted barn. Glasgow/Essex: disparity in wealth, disparity in opportunity. What was happening to Britain in 1987? What was happening to Scotland, to England?

Many years later I learn that the Sandoz family own the

Beau-Rivage. Didn't they once make LSD? Later I also learn about the No Free Lunch movement, medics against what they perceive as the sometimes-malign influence of pharmaceutical companies on drug purchasing and prescribing decisions. Since Lausanne I've felt a bit queasy around Big Pharma and its manipulations. Check out the recent OxyContin/Purdue Pharma scandal...

Returning to the north side of the Clyde it was part of my job to do a formal teaching session once a week. This meant identifying a patient with a good story, an interesting history; drawing up seven seats around their bed; getting the students to sit in a semi-circle once the screens were drawn; and encouraging them to tease out the patient's experience. I particularly enjoyed chatting with a Mr Ronald Borland.

Ronald was a fisherman from the Outer Hebrides, from South Uist to be precise. I'd visited the island with my wife not long before meeting Ronald and loved its solitude, its stark beauty and its pristine white empty beaches. Ronald flew down to Glasgow once a month for a procedure called plasmapheresis: essentially a process where his blood was put through a washing machine. He had noticed a tremor in his hands six months previously and Moira, my senior colleague, herself an islander from nearby Benbecula, had identified that his Parkinsonian signs were the result of a rare condition called Waldenstrom's macroglobulinaemia; two more great words. She wrote up the case and got it published. Ronald was making too much of a protein called immunoglobulin M, which increased the viscosity of his blood, thickening it, and causing him to have small strokes that rendered him Parkinsonian. The wash would, theoretically, prevent him having any more of these.

Each time I saw Ronald I'd be impressed by his quiet patience, his stoicism. He had a weather-beaten face from his time sailing on the Minch and his voice was soft and mellifluous, a beguiling trait most of the islanders share. I'd ask how was life on South Uist and he'd always reply that it was beautiful, that the weather had been marvellous and the fishing good. He was brave: he was a real old man of the sea. Ronald spoke of the eternal verities in plain language: the first, but not the last, truly Hemingway-esque person I would meet in my career.

Jane was another of the regulars we taught on. She had long-standing Type 1 diabetes and now that she was in her thirties she was running into deep trouble. A small but persistent number of young people like Jane with insulin-dependent diabetes find it very hard to come to terms with the diagnosis. As a result, she had been admitted to hospital almost weekly for ten years or more. Jane had had thousands of admissions. Her case notes came in several thick volumes. I think she was on volume eight when I knew her. By the time she died you could have stacked her notes in a tower and found that they were taller than you were.

By omitting her insulin, she would go into ketoacidosis, a condition that, to this day, has a 10 per cent mortality rate. I'd first come across ketoacidosis in an Alistair MacLean novel called *Night Without End* I'd read as a boy. A plane crashes in the Arctic wastes (something to do with the CIA or the KGB, I recall, but isn't that always the case with MacLean?) and one of the passengers has diabetes and runs out of insulin. They will die soon if not rescued. There was a detail that caught my childhood attention and that I have long remembered: the breath of this passenger began to smell sweet, like pear drops or nail varnish remover. This was the scent of acetone, a ketone body, a chemical the body makes if it can no longer utilise glucose through the lack of insulin. This was not the sweet smell of success but the smell of imminent death. You could often tell Jane was on the ward before you left the nursing station. You could smell the pear drops.

Ketoacidosis is treated with intravenous fluids and insulin. This means access: venous access. But after a thousand admissions and a thousand attacks on her veins Jane had run out of obvious places to insert a line. Jane's hands, her feet, her elbow hollows, all the veins you would expect to find there had all thrombosed, closed down into thick ropes of scar tissue. These were impossible to cannulate. To compound matters Jane was overweight and this made the access problem even more acute.

She ate sweets and rubbish all the time, part of her psychological coping mechanism. Her bedside locker was littered with Bounty wrappers, Mars bars, bags of those pink-coloured pear drop boilings, *just in case I go hypo*. In case her blood sugar went low. And to be fair to her you really did not want Jane to go hypoglycaemic: trying to correct hypoglycaemia by injecting her with hyper-viscous 50 per cent dextrose was damn near impossible.

You had to ask yourself how awful someone's home circumstances have to be in order to prefer admission to hospital to trying to cope in the outside world. I would learn that many of these youngsters had a quite horrific home life, their parents abusive or in jail. The children would stop giving themselves insulin because the only love they knew, the etiolated version of love they got in hospital, was, for them, infinitely better than their traumatic existence outside.

The anaesthetists had been called in countless times to cannulate Jane's central veins, these being behind the clavicle that led directly to the heart. Now even these were roped off. We needed a long-term plan or she would die. Kris was on the case. He came up with the idea of a pump.

No ordinary pump: the external ones that had just come on the market were proving rather unpopular in those early days of pump technology. They would break down, leading the patient to come back in again with another life-threatening episode of ketoacidosis. Jane had tried an external pump, but we were pretty sure she was disconnecting it when she got home. Kris scoured the medical journals and found an answer. There was a man in Austria who had developed a new type of pump. So Kris took her to Vienna. There she would have an internal pump inserted in her chest wall: a subcutaneous pump that would connect to one of the few veins centrally that remained patent.

Jane was ecstatic when she returned. For an all-too-brief spell her emergency hospital admissions stopped. She had to pop up to the ward every two weeks, however, to have her pump filled with insulin. I couldn't help noticing how she would often gravitate towards some other young patients in nearby beds. I'd overhear her giving them some bad piece of advice. She was perpetuating her own conflicts and, perhaps inadvertently, encouraging others to go down the same troubled road she had travelled. I've seen very many versions of Jane since and, sadly, most met premature ends.

A decade or so later my new team would get to know another girl with problems just like Jane's. She was admitted weekly for a period of at least five years with episodes of ketoacidosis. Her mother was in jail. Her father was an alcoholic, her brother feral. Her life was a Randy Newman song without the irony, a Tom Waits dirge without the possibility of redemption. She just got sicker and sicker as the years passed. And then, bizarrely, she won the National Lottery: tens of thousands of pounds. Amazingly she also conceived and had a relatively healthy pregnancy despite her appalling diabetes control. She died of overwhelming sepsis and kidney failure a few years back, well short of her fortieth birthday, her child not yet in double figures.

To fill Jane's pump, you had to palpate the thick disc that had been implanted under her skin, an object the size of a puck – that's what her pump looked like, an ice-hockey puck. With a gloved finger you had to press down on her skin above the pump to find a tiny central depression where a rubber entrance point could be probed by a needle. It was hard not to think about darts, Jim Bowen and *Bullseye*. Once in (*you've won the speedboat!*) you then connected the needle to a giving set, some plastic tubes that led in turn to a large syringe that contained Jane's two-week supply of insulin. Every fortnight the pump had to be filled.

I remember that we then had to connect the apparatus to a syringe driver, a hand-cranked piece of Heath Robinson technology that was a beast to turn. Kris was expert at manipulating this gizmo.

Kris's fellow SR, Martin, was a driven young man from the poorer east end of the city. Like Kris, he had a verbal tic: it was Kris who said *absolutely* all the time; Martin, *hi team!* We shared teaching duties with Kris and Martin and Simon. Simon was another SR, an expert on bone. Simon was dishevelled, scatty, his hair always awry, but he was very, very bright. All three could relate to the punters and it was easy to identify with them, to want to emulate them. They had none of the stand-offish character that possessed some on the west side of the city.

I watched Simon teach one day. He put an arm around an old lady who sat on a bed and then turned to the students and said: 'Always try to keep some eye contact with the patient.'

He then turned to the old soul, still in his clutches, and stared into her eyes like some demented hypnotist, like a mad Dr Mabuse figure. He addressed the students again, his first two fingers making a flicking gesture from his eyes to hers: 'You'll be watched closely by the examiners as you examine. So remember… always give it the caring jazz.'

I see Simon's face now, his fake smile flashing at the gobsmacked patient, and his insouciant hand-gesturing. I still hear his explicitly cynical exposure: the truth, the rules of the game. I laughed in shock at his blatant indifference to our surprise. Why was I astonished? Simon was an actor revealing the secrets of our craft. Medicine *is* something of an act. We have to be distanced or else we might crack up, burst out crying on ward rounds. Which would be no good for anyone. Medicine is about calming patients with their Nabokovian 'controlled panic'. Our job is to try to ameliorate this with our controlled pity. *Always give it the caring jazz.*

I note that after Oliver Sacks finished his own teaching sessions he would break with the students for some tea, but it was coffee for us, always coffee. An integral part of the whole doctoring experience is a constant topping-up with harsh cups of Nescafé, none of that ground Yemeni hipster five quid a cup stuff. Sacks goes on to say that 'weather permitting, we might go across to the New York Botanical Garden, where we would settle under a tree and talk about philosophy and life generally'. Uh, we didn't do that over coffee in Glasgow.

Our conversations were more Brian Cant than Immanuel Kant. We gabbed and reminisced about kids' shows like *Trumpton*. These ad-hoc symposia were held in a grotty canteen that served bridies. The weather permitted nothing.

Sacks was brilliant, but I have long noted his apparent ability to avoid the daily grind, the front door. Sacks knew about causality but not *Casualty*. I cannot imagine working with him. Fascinating his case histories may be, but Sacks reminds me powerfully of a few doctors I've worked with: the ones who find it a struggle to see more than two patients of an afternoon. Managers would be on Sacks's case very sharply these days. Essentially Sacks was a stamp-collector. His cases were the Penny Blacks, the Inverted Jennys, of medicine. He knew, rightly, that patients and their stories made for great literary vignettes. But there's always the suspicion he tended to savour the more freakish conditions. He's the Barnum of medicine. *Look what this guy can't do!* There is an inescapable hint of voyeuristic glee in his descriptions, as if he were holding each patient delicately up to the light with a pair of tweezers for our delectation: *check that watermark.*

For all the fine words said about his sensitivity and caring, my suspicion is that Sacks would have done almost anything to avoid the really tough stuff, the A+E madness, the busy epilepsy clinics. Anything routine. All a bit beneath him, one suspects. Not enough fascinating overprints, interrupted perforations or, even better, imperforations; the imperfections he loved to collect. Sharing a rota with Oliver Sacks would have been an unpredictable source of dread: when would I have to cover him? As the years practising pass I find myself increasingly, irrationally, crabby with Sacks and asking this as I enviously see piles of his books: exactly how many nights did he *actually* do on call in his life? How often did he get out of bed at two in the morning?

I worked out after I retired that I did more than a thousand nights on call. More than three years of an entire life spent on call. Beat you at that, Oliver, if nothing else. But I have to face it: that guy taught me more than most.

Celebrity doctors are somewhat distrusted in the profession because they often exceed their brief; they prattle on about conditions they have had no real experience of dealing with. Tele-doctors seem to be selected on the basis of their physical attractiveness and erotic unattainability. Print docs relish their relative anonymity and often use pseudonyms. Those who write for the more outrageous right-wing magazines have been prone to bullying snobberies – that and frank racism. Some love to prime the public in panic.

I once wrote to one such doctor who was quoted in one of the dailies as saying that you could get diabetes from sitting exams. I asked him where did he get this information from and he quoted a paper, apparently published in Nebraska, an obscure journal with a low impact factor. 'Impact factor' is the gauge used by academics to assess the importance of a paper. Getting in the *New England Journal of Medicine* has a high impact factor. Maybe the newspaper's top doc was playing a gag on me, one worthy of a medical version of Mark Twain. I couldn't find any references from Nebraska; there was no smoking gun in Omaha. Did he make up that tall tale about diabetes and exams? As Twain once said: never let the truth stand in the way of a good story.

Teaching with an actual patient meant unprecedented access into the interiority of said individual. This I tried to stress to the students. Try to find out what the patient has done in their life. You will be constantly surprised. Those who had survived the Second World War were particularly fascinating. I recall a conversation with a regal old lady on a ward round when the students were present. After we had examined her abdomen (she had inflamed gallstones but the surgeons were not interested, hence her being under us; surgical resistance is a recurrent theme in the life of physicians) I asked: 'So, did you work during the war then?'

'I did, yes. I was in West Africa.'

'Really?' and then the inevitable: 'Where?'

'Sierra Leone.'

'Right.'

I hesitate and then ask archly: 'And did you meet a Mr Greene there?'

She's coy but answers slowly, suspiciously: 'I did, yes.'

I know the conversation has to change direction now. Her discretion is signalled with great dignity. Her eyes say: *Do not ask me any more*. She has signed the Official Secrets Act.

Later, over coffee with the students, I asked if they knew what the lady had been, what her job was. They sat blankly. I told them: 'She was a spy. She worked with Graham Greene.'

But they were not as impressed as I'd hoped. They hadn't heard of Greene.

'*The Heart of the Matter? The Power and the Glory?*'

Shakes of the head.

'*Brighton Rock*, surely.'

Some vague nods. In the twenty-first century I would sit with one student who, after a conversation about dictators, asked me who Stalin was.

Polish patients of a certain age were always interesting. If they told me that they had come over in 1939 I'd ask if they had served in the RAF. I could then nod to the students and tell them later that the frail old gentleman they had just met with pneumonia had probably fought in the Battle of Britain. And if they had come over in 1946 then, over coffee again, I'd ask the students what they knew about war criminals. I'd ask what would they think if one of the patients they had to look after was in fact an old SS man? What would they do if one night they were asked to care for the wounds of an ISIS bomber? Would they look after a terrorist?

Cue furrowed foreheads, some backchat and a bit of the old dialectics.

Philosophy in the Botanical Gardens with Dr Sacks: that must have been nice. I wonder if Sacks sneaked in some references to Theodor Adorno or Hannah Arendt over sips of tea. I bet he did. Even if I suspect he was work-shy I'm jealous of his students. I would love to have been one. I see they've now even named a planet after him.

My dad called me one night many years later when I was a consultant and asked if I'd looked after a certain Mr F he had been reading about. So I said yes I had, he was under my care, and my dad asked if I'd known that this man was the world expert on German photography. He'd written the definitive book on the subject and my dad had just read his obituary. Shamed, I said no. Mr F had been under my care for only a few days and I didn't know this. I hadn't asked him what he had done with his life.

As a registrar, I was allowed to teach much more now – which would also, of course, involve lecturing. Lecturing is notoriously tricky. There was a study published that looked at the duration of attention span during lectures which showed that most people switch off after about five minutes. Lecturers need to use tactics to keep an audience alert, to switch them on and then on again, to continually reboot them. Like a stand-up comedian, I thought. You need to watch stand-up comedians to know how to keep an audience enthralled. You need to learn from them how to keep the students awake. I honed my act, even if I wasn't a fuckin' comedian.

But lecturing could afford the chance to have wild flights of fancy, flights that soared as crazily as a kid threatening a jumbo jet with a drone. Endocrinologists have always been fascinated by the interaction of a hormone and its receptor, not unlike a key and a lock, this being a useful analogy when explaining problems to a patient. Textbooks and PowerPoint presentations usually illustrate this interaction with a drawing of *one* hormone and *one* receptor, one key and one lock, resembling two interlocking pieces of Lego. I could mentally fly trying to explain this.

I would delight in drawing the students' attention to the carpet on the lecture hall floor. This had a closely knit pixelated-like pattern. I'd ask the audience to imagine that the floor was a gigantically enlarged surface of one cell and that each of these pixels was a receptor, a lock. So there were hundreds of thousands of receptors, locks, on just one cell surface and then I'd ask them to imagine (my arms flying hither and thither above the carpet) hundreds and thousands of hormones, keys, landing on each of these receptors, locks, and all interacting in different concentrations at any given time. And if that concept weren't mind-blowing enough I'd ask them to now picture life *under* the carpet, maybe ten feet below us (my arms now making an underground digging gesture like The Spinners doing 'Working My Way Back to You') to where the cell nucleus resided. The cell nucleus received all the messages after the keys had unlocked, then synthesised them and decided what the overall story it was getting from the surface was and acted accordingly.

These cells were from all over the body, everywhere: did they know that the gut was an endocrine organ? That even their lowly colons were endocrine organs sending messages to the brain? And that boring old white fat tissue was an endocrine organ, that the heart, yeah, even the heart, had an endocrine function? Go tell those fancy cool cat cardiologists that. If this were not enough (making a face that read: *far out, man!*) there was that ten-foot gap between the carpet and the nucleus which was filled with thousands of post-receptor signalling messages, any one of which might be faulty or have a mutation and... and... and. At that point I'd pause and ask: how could they *not* want to become an endocrinologist?

William Blake's idea of heaven in a wildflower. He was right: another heaven in the universe is the endocrinology of just one cell.

Despite the prodigious feats of memory that medical students are asked to complete, usually in the second year at university, learning the names of every nerve, muscle, artery and so on in anatomy, I was always amazed at how much of this information they had contrived to forget by the time they were halfway through their third year. And so, when I would revise the cranial nerves with the students it would quickly become apparent how many had forgotten them. There are twelve. However, cut them some slack: how many of the twelve Apostles can you name? Go on, try. And so we would go back to a mnemonic, a word I always stumbled in pronouncing. Was it mem–nun–ick? Muh–nem–nun–ick? I'd fantasise aloud that in time the only thing they would remember of my teaching was this inability. *Do you remember that guy that used to teach us the cranial nerves, the guy who couldn't pronounce mnemonic?*

The mnemonic for the cranial nerves begins: 'Oh, oh, oh, to tickle and fondle.' Olfactory, optic, oculomotor, trochlear, facial. *Fondle!* Or was it feel? No kidding: this is what generations of medical students in the UK have been taught. And the rest of the mnemonic would go on to mention virgins and hymens and God knows what else. The students would laugh. I'd then particularly address the women in the group and say, with disdain: 'Look, it's now the twenty-first century and you guys (*guys*, it was always guys when talking to the collective; I'd quickly registered the frowns when I used the word 'girls' early in the new century) have had feminism and post-feminism and equal rights and the feminisation of the work force and all that and yet you still remember the cranial nerves with this sexist rubbish of a muh-nem-nun-ick about virginity.'

So I'd urge them to ensure that the famed mnemonic for the cranial nerves is condemned to the dumpster of history as soon as possible. Incidentally, going back to the twelve Apostles, you forgot Thaddeus, right?

We would move on and I'd go round the room asking each student in turn to list the nerves, one through twelve, as I wrote the names on a flip-chart with one of those lime-green or blood-red marker pens that would inevitably smear your fingers for the rest of the working afternoon. Number one was olfactory and we would digress (it was difficult to avoid digression but I'd learned that digression, seemingly chaotic digression, was the way to maintain attention, make the student unclear of what might happen next) about how a perfumer with a head injury damaging their olfactory nerve might lose their job, or a sommelier maybe.

We would then spend some more time over number two, the optic nerve, and here I would fake visual field deficits: a homonymous hemianopia or a bitemporal hemianopia, and get them to practise testing on each other, again a technique to prevent boredom. You compare your field of vision in one eye with that of the patient or student opposite, all the while both of you trying to fix your gaze forward, covering one eye with one hand and using the other hand to wiggle fingers and map any field defect temporally, i.e. outwards. *Tell me when you can see my finger.* This would often end in hilarity as some of them had an inability to wink, an essential skill when comparing your own *nasal* visual field with a patient's, that is to say seeing inwards towards your nose. If you could not wink then you found your arms tangling up like the tentacles of a drunken octopus.

I'd often go on about how the brain, the occipital lobe, corrects the image on the retina by turning it right side up. But does that mean that reality was upside down? More cod-philosophy, imagining I'd somehow graduated from the school of Sacks. Then another digression: did any of them ever lie on the ground as a kid and stare at the sky and imagine that the sky was really the earth and that they were flying way, way high above it? Why don't they go out this weekend if the weather was good and do that again? Just take a day out and lie on the ground and stare at the clouds and the sky. I'd register their scepticism and move on.

I could not fake problems with cranial nerves numbers three, four and six: respectively the oculomotor, trochlear and abducens nerves. Palsies of these nerves cause double vision, diplopia and non-conjugate movements of the eyes. Some *real* comedians can or could do this trick: I have a memory of an exophthalmic Marty Feldman – the Igor figure in *Young Frankenstein* – doing very odd things with his eyes. Marty had had terrible thyroid eye disease: in time I'd come across a few similar cases.

Nerves five and seven are, respectively, the nerves of facial sensation and expression. I'd get the group to shut their eyes tightly, frown, smile and blow out their cheeks, all ways of revealing a facial palsy and how you can discriminate between one that has been caused by a Bell's palsy (complete paralysis of one side of the face) and one caused by a stroke (the patient can still frown).

Eight, vestibulocochlear, involved twanging a tuning fork and placing it behind the ear. Nine is glossopharyngeal and involves staring at the uvula. I'd digress again and go on about my wife and how she once mistook an advert for a Batman movie at a bus shelter for an intraoral view of the uvula. She just couldn't see it: like that famed rabbit/duck illusion.

Ten was vagus and for stupid reasons I'd always sing the line 'Viva

Las Vegas' in a bad impression of Elvis. Vagus was great because you could skip right past it: bedside testing was not particularly helpful. Eleven, accessory, meant shrugging the shoulders and turning the neck against force. Twelve, hypoglossal, meant sticking out your tongue. And that was that. I'd maybe conclude by saying something like: 'Relax. The neurologists will go through this again with you. They'll take out little pins to map the visual field and little bottles to test taste and smell – but in real life you'll have no more than five minutes to check the average patient's cranial nerves.'

I could see their faces silently incredulous asking: *five minutes*?

'You will be in A+E with the crowds waiting to be seen so you'll need to master a quick examination of the cranial nerves. You need to get your examination technique down pat. On a busy day you will have no more than one hour to see someone, get their story, examine them, order the tests. That means you need to do the cranial nerves in five minutes flat. Now, let's practise again.'

Sometimes I'd enjoy a deranged rant as a way of keeping them engaged, alert. When talking at our next session on the neurology of the arm and hand, I'd go on about the opponens muscles in the thumb. We would get on to talking about monkeys and how they can't oppose thumb and finger. I'd bang on about how I hated monkeys (not true) and how in the zoo they would shit and masturbate and stare at you insolently but that my advice was to stare them out and slowly, very slowly, show them how you could oppose thumb and finger. Give them an anatomical lesson in superiority that says: sod you. *You can't do this.*

I would impersonate a satisfied diner when I was teaching about the arm. We would discuss how a shoulder dystocia, a birth where the shoulder is difficult to deliver, might result in something called an Erb's palsy. The palsy is also known as a waiter's tip deformity.

I'd demonstrate what the waiter's tip deformity looked like: a sur-
reptitious backhanded gesture. But I'd strongly advise them *against*
tipping like this in some far-off future.

I'd rant too about my time at school and confess my insensitivities as a kid and how schoolmates would bully the afflicted merci-
lessly, like our teacher Dan who had an Erb's palsy. We called him
'Para Handy' after a Scottish TV character. Then there was the time
in first year at secondary school when I heard some sideline wags
watching others play football. They were shouting to a boy with
hydrocephalus (fluid on the brain): 'Heid!' *Heeeed the baw.* They
called this poor big lad with the poor big head he was born with
'Heid': '*Heid that baw, Heid.*'

And yet at the same time the kids at my school were surprisingly
kind to a wee lad with phocomelia. His vestigial arms were seal-like
flippers (seal-like hence 'phoco') and were the drastically horrific
result of that most terrible of 1960s pharmaceutical scandals: the
thalidomide affair.

I'm back with the students on another session and teaching the
muscles of the leg. We would get on to an odd one called 'sartorius'.
I would discuss the etymology of the term and go on about Savile
Row tailors and suits, hence sartorial. Tailors were said to balance
rolls of cloth with the use of the sartorius muscle by flexing their leg
just so. I'd demonstrate standing like a stork. Sometimes of a bored
weekend I'd pop my head into Moss Bros or some other high street
tailor and pose at the doorway by flexing my leg into said position,
and when accosted by the sales people simply point at my contor-
tion, smile and say: 'Sartorius, eh? Brilliant muscle.'

I didn't. I never did this. My wife cringes when I tell her this story.
But, as a way of avoiding boredom, it was fun to see if the students
believed me.

Inspired by Sacks, I'd get the students to fake the various types of tremor, the different types of gait, and ask them to imagine what it must be like to have one of these disabilities *all the time*. I'd make them walk the length of a room with the swinging circumduction gait of a patient with a stroke, the arm often held over the chest flexed in spasticity. Or ask them to festinate (beautiful word), to chase the centre of their body's gravity in the shuffling steps that can afflict the Parkinsonian patient. In doing this perhaps for a few seconds they could imagine the horror of living with such a challenge. Then to distract I'd usually ask the students if they knew the meaning of the word 'festinate'. One time a lad asked if it was something to do with windows. Eh? No, but a good try. This led to a discussion about windows and being chucked out of windows. Which led on to defenestration and Czech revolutionaries and Prague and how someone festinating might be at increased risk of defenestration. Especially if you were in Prague: never festinate near a window in Prague.

We were acting then. John Berger describes the country doctor John Sassall in his beautiful book *A Fortunate Man* this way: 'If you met him outside his area, on neutral ground, and if he didn't begin talking, you might for one moment suppose that he was an actor. He might have been one. In this way too he would have played many roles.'

What are those roles we play as doctors? Priest, teacher, politician, leader, Master Mariner, entertainer, comedian. Comedian? Make 'em laugh. Sassall was a GP in the Forest of Dean: a very different life from mine. My patients had eight fingers, his thirteen.

Sassall's way of living, his choice of specialty in general practice, reminds me of a Friday evening in the mid-1980s when I had to do a talk in Newcastle. I jumped into my car with a blue box full of slides and tore down south. The abandoned factories and depots of the city soon gave way to the bleak uplands. And then as England neared the land became greener, prettier: I was in the Borders. Thirsty, I stopped off in Jedburgh to buy a can of cola and, time against me, jogged towards a small confectionery shop. And there, standing patiently waiting to be served, was a guy who qualified at the same time as me, a guy in my year.

He was the local GP and he was proudly wearing a Barbour jacket and wellington boots. He held a dog on a leash. A gun dog in memory, but then I'm now arming him with a shotgun over his elbow and a deerstalker on his head like Thomas Gainsborough's Mr Andrews. I'm pretty sure he didn't have any of these on board, but you get the picture. Now I'm standing there catching my breath after scooting over from the car park, Marks & Spencer cheap suit on as ever, scuffed sensible shoes. I'm in a hurry; he is not. I'm still chasing some sort of career certitude; his is now fixed, he has tenure. I'm urban; he is rural. I want to be thought a serious person in the city; he is happy to be important in his modest small town. He is content. I am ego-driven, still hustling. We stare at one another and smile in recognition and then talk. When we part, we shake hands: we have each made our choice and we are both sure of our decision. We are in different roles. He is a patient man: I am not.

I could never have been a GP.

I read another phrase from Berger about a patient who has come to see Dr Sassall: 'She was still young enough for her face to change totally with her expression.' This is a good and simple observation about age and ageing. But I think James Kennaway bests this with another, crueller phrase from his novel *Some Gorgeous Accident*: 'Age was chasing sex from her face.' He means gender. As with old hirsute ladies or old feminised men (like those with prostate cancer on testosterone blockers). Genderless faces: the ones most of us end up having. This saddens me: again the need to control pity.

Another busy night on call. Ward Seven is the admissions ward: this is where patients are transferred after a preliminary assessment in A+E. Ward Seven is where we get a better picture of what's really going on with the sick, where we review all the investigations, where the complexities of disease are revealed. There are many single rooms to help us isolate someone if necessary – if, say, there is any question of an infective disease. The sisters and nurses on the ward are all highly experienced and are diplomatically skilled at steering doctors when they might be heading in the wrong direction. They are not afraid of pushing us physically to see someone quickly if needs be. They have scissors at the ready; stitching kits; those polished silver metal trays with drapes for doing lumbar punctures, sigmoidoscopies and chest drains. They have iodine packs so that we can turn snow-white swabs the colour of burnt toffee. They are ready to bring a crashing fist down on a stopped heart.

One of the sisters is very worried about a young girl in a side room. I've worked with this sister for four years now and know that she has a sixth sense. Many talented nurses have this: in addition to their superhuman empathy and patience they can smell trouble. She blows some strands of hair that have fallen over her brow and swears casually, but then we all do that here in this war zone: 'She's fucked, JDQ. You'd better see her ASAP.'

So I dash into the young girl's side room and see immediately that the sister is right. The kid is sweating profusely and is pale; she's as white as her sheets. I recall JBF talking to an anaemic patient once. He lifted his palm high and said in a Tonto accent: 'How, paleface!'

There's no time for joking with this kid, though; she is dying in front of my eyes: 'What have A+E said is wrong with her?'

The sister wipes her brow and is quick in replying: 'Pneumothorax.'

God, how I hate pneumothoraxes. I'm like Indiana Jones with

the Nazis: I hate these guys. A pneumothorax: air in the chest cavity compressing the lungs. I might have to stick an emergency chest drain into the kid. Shit. Drains are vicious things: sticking a drain in is a controlled form of stabbing. Stabbing someone in the chest. And it doesn't look as if we have much time to wait for local anaesthetic to work. This will be brutal. I've heard stories of doctors going too far south with the drain and puncturing the heart itself. Doctors have killed people with chest drains. I flick the stethoscope dangling around my neck and plug it in my ears and listen to the girl's chest. I listen in as carefully, as intently, as Olivier Messiaen must have listened to birdsong maybe, or as John Cage did to silence, and can clearly hear breath sounds on both sides. I'm certain of this. I'd swear to this. I can hear an inspiratory sniff, an expiratory sigh. On both sides. I am not hearing silence. Silence equals a big pneumothorax. Silence equals get out the chest drain, get out the iodine swabs, get ready to stab.

So I figure… if she does have a pneumothorax then it can't be a big one. It can't be making her this unwell. The sister switches on the light box in the room and I thrust the chest X-ray up against it with that always-pleasing *thunk* sound as the metal surround grabs the film. I stare at the monochrome image and see a very small apical pneumothorax on the right (thank you God that it's not on the left: there's little risk of inadvertent cardiac puncture now) and think: That can't be making her *this* sick. Something else is going on. I don't think she is septic; she doesn't have a temperature. She looks like she's bleeding. She has the terminally grey colour you see when someone is vomiting up buckets of blood from ruptured varices. She denies vomiting when I ask her. She hasn't lost blood from anywhere obvious either. She's just about conscious. I squint up at the X-ray again and note on the right-hand side there is also a small amount of fluid present at her lung base. An effusion. I listen to her chest again and percuss: yes, she is dull to percussion at that right base. What the fuck is going on? I'll phone JBF. He hears the story and his calmness reassures me. He's quick to diagnose the problem: 'I think she must be bleeding into her chest, JDQ. She's got a haemopneumothorax.'

A haemopneumothorax? A *spontaneous* haemopneumothorax! Is there such a thing? Does that even *happen*? I've never even heard of this happening. Was it in the textbooks? If it was no one taught us about it. *No one has EVER told us about this!* I want to shout out loud to the ward, the hospital, the High Street and the Manx bar, the Merchant City and the world: I HAVE NOT BEEN TAUGHT ABOUT THIS!

I think to myself: If this does turn out to be a haemopneumothorax then it must be helluva rare. Is it? And then I think JBF is some man if he has got this right over the phone. She must be bleeding for no apparent reason into her chest; I know from the blood tests that her clotting is reassuringly normal.

I call the cardiothoracic guys, who descend on us and take her to theatre with speed, where, with transfusions, she is operated on and survives.

I'm appalled by the randomness of this event. The universe and its laws have thrown this girl (and me too) a nasty curveball. This is small-print stuff. This is not what you need on a night when the ward is swarming with alcoholics screaming nonsense at you about beasties crawling up and down the wall. In acute withdrawal, the jakeys in delirium tremens, they've got shivers down the backbone; they've got the shaking all over. Like some William Burroughs nightmare, the ward is crawling with junkies demanding methadone: *Just gie us some, Doc, gie us some methadone tae get us aff the junk.*

'Common things occur commonly': that's one of the mantras you hear constantly in medicine, in A+E, in the admissions wards, but uncommon things can happen too. Rare events occur and that is when you may need to call up the seniors with their twenty or thirty years' experience ahead of you.

But what if they don't know either? Then you go ever higher. Who and where is our peak opinion? Our Ben Nevis, our Everest? As a doctor you will find yourself asking: 'Who would know more about this condition, who is the best opinion in Britain, in Europe, in America, on the planet?' And then you get on the phone and *phone* them.

8

BOBBY

Dr Hastie introduces me to Bobby. He's a ten-year-old kid: that's way outside our usual comfort zone as adult physicians. Problem is the paediatricians don't know what to do with him. Bobby is small for his age and has thick dark hair set on a low brow that helmets his face. He has rough brown patches on his skin around his flexures, his elbows; his neck looks as if it needs a good scrub, but this I know is another sign, a skin sign, called acanthosis nigricans. And this sign implies insulin resistance. Insulin as a key, the receptor as a lock: Bobby has plenty of keys but not enough locks. This is why the paediatricians aren't winning. Bobby has been referred to us because his insulin receptors are not working.

Insulin receptors sit on the cell surface and, just as you need a key and a lock to get in a door, if you have no key (no insulin) then you are in trouble. No key and you have Type 1 diabetes; you need insulin, you need insulin *fast*. If you have no locks, however, then no matter how much insulin your body makes it cannot get the cell to act. Then you are in real trouble: effectively you are like one of those unfortunates with Type 1 diabetes before 1922, before insulin was discovered. Look at the old black and white pictures: desperate parents cradling a thin, wasted child. Skin and bones. They all died before insulin was discovered in Canada. This is what Bobby faced. Globally, every year since God knows when, hundreds of thousands of people went into ketoacidosis and died. They still do in the poorer parts of Africa without insulin.

The paediatricians have asked us if we have any ideas. Kris and Dr Hastie have one, a great idea: they are thinking about another hormone altogether, a substance called IGF-1. Insulin-like growth factor 1. As it says on the tin, IGF-1 is *insulin-like*. And it is known to lower blood sugar levels in rats if you give it to them intravenously. IGF-1 does this by acting through its *own* receptor, its own lock. So our plan is to bypass Bobby's faulty insulin receptor. We are pretty sure Bobby has IGF receptors because if he hadn't then he would have died shortly after birth. But it has never been used before in humans. And where would we get it from anyway?

Japan.

Dr Hastie and I arrange to meet up with some of the drug company people from Osaka. When they fly over, the meeting resembles all those clichéd East–West encounters that Hollywood enjoys mocking: like Bill Murray in *Lost in Translation* we stumble verbally over one another after the mutual bowing and handshakes. We stress the danger Bobby is in, the extreme urgency of the situation. We think that when he hits puberty his insulin resistance will be exacerbated. This happens in kids with Type 1 diabetes.

Our accents and rapid diction notwithstanding, some sense is achieved and we get an agreement: we will ask for ethical committee approval to try IGF-1 with Bobby, and the Japanese will supply the drug.

We speak to Bobby's parents. His mum is sparky, determined and has a need for knowledge; she wants us to do everything we can. His dad is a quiet, hard-working man, a stoic; his face lined and sad-dened by his son's suffering. They are fully aware that Bobby is close to death. They know that the chances of success are slim, but they are willing to try anything. And Bobby himself? He's a bright lad with a talent for drawing Disney-style cartoons and he entertains the nurses with his practical jokes. Today there would be no way he'd be placed in an adult ward, but my memory is that the other patients, the hemiplegic cases, the terminally ill, were, if anything, cheered by his presence. The paediatric hospital was on the other side of the city and it was impractical to see him there daily.

It's my job to talk to Bobby, to gain his trust, his confidence. I have a brother his age and so I'm used to talking about kids' TV shows and cartoon characters. Over on the female ward Kris is still cranking up the pump for Jane. The team has decided: Bobby is my charge.

We need blood and poor Bobby has had a bucket taken from him over the years. He's brave and lets us puncture his leathery skin and get some samples off to the lab. Our colleague in Cambridge, an Irish genius called Steve O'Rahilly, analyses some samples we send down and confirms the drastic nature of Bobby's insulin resistance. Steve agrees with our plan to try IGF-1; he will be a constant source of encouragement and support. The vials of IGF-1 arrive from Japan and each small bottle contains a wad of drug that resembles a plastic washer. This must be dissolved in water before we inject. Each sample costs God knows how many yen.

No one has ever given the drug to a human before. I draw it up. We have an array of bottles at his bedside, a syringe of glucose drawn up in case his sugars dive, in case he goes profoundly hypoglycaemic. Profound hypoglycaemia can be fatal.

I've spoken to Bobby again and we have discussed the plan

carefully with his parents. The cannula, the Venflon, pink, one of the smallest, sits in a vein on the back of his hand. I ask Bobby if he's ready and he says yes. I inject and I'm aware of my own pulse racing. He laughs as I take a deep breath. And then he says to me: 'There, that wasn't so bad, was it?'

He is aware how much I fear a bad outcome. But the blood sugar levels, remarkably, fall. The IGF-1 has worked through his own IGF receptors and bypassed the faulty insulin receptor. He's alive and has not gone hypoglycaemic either: a world first.

But this is no Banting and Best moment: this is not like the discovery of insulin; this is no miracle cure for diabetes. For one, the condition that Bobby has (known as the Rabson-Mendenhall syndrome) is astonishingly rare. In consequence, the Japanese know that any commercial value for IGF-1 is likely to be extremely limited. And we are not at all sure on dosages, on how often we should give the drug, on what side effects (apart from hypoglycaemia) we should watch out for.

Bobby is remarkably patient. He is tearful sometimes when he needs a new cannula, but he soon picks up and then bounces around the ward showing Dr Hastie his caricatures of Kris, of Dr Hastie himself, of me. And we get him home.

His mum and dad are aware that although the blood sugars are better the IGF-1 is no cure. At best it will be like insulin itself, *insulin-like*, something that will keep him alive but will not necessarily prevent complications. I look after Bobby for three years or more and then leave the city, move south as JBF predicted, and come to London. The team at King's is keen to know more about our use of IGF-1.

I hear three years later from Glasgow that Bobby's condition is worsening, that he is getting serious infections that are proving deep-seated. He's tiring. I speak with his mum and dad on the phone. And then Bobby dies. I head up and see him in his small coffin. And I think of all those other brave patients who, although long dead, have enlightened medicine through their own experiences, their own sufferings, who have benefited mankind but who are not remembered. I want Bobby remembered.

Bobby and his practical jokes: syringes filled with water that he would use as pistols; cling film over toilet seats.

Practical jokes are OK if you're a kid. But not if you're an adult: practical jokes are juvenile. Adults should not play practical jokes. You're not a fuckin' comedian. So why did I play one on Danvers?

Danvers had recovered from his angry confrontation with the anaesthetist at that torrid cardiac arrest. He was a cardiology registrar now in the land of pacing wires and coronary angiography, the land of Hutchinson with his third and fourth heart *soinds*. Danvers and his wife were due over at our house one night for dinner. The night they were due round I somehow noticed that Kylie Minogue was playing at one of the city's venues. Kylie may have been cute and camp, kitsch and popular, but I knew neither Danvers nor I were particularly interested in her music. Or so I guessed. I'm still not sure what possessed me, but I reached for the phone and bleeped him via the switchboard. And when he answered I put on an Australian accent, Strine, secure in the knowledge that he would see through the joke immediately: 'Hello, is that yer Dr Poole, Dr Danvers Poole?'

He answers 'yes' suspiciously. I keep up the Strine: 'My name is Lance Ritchie and I'm phoning you from yer Australian consulate, down in yer Nelson Mandela Square. Love you Glasgow guys for calling it that: can you speak, mate?'

Again, a hesitant voice that answers formally in his best authoritative doctoring tone: 'Yes, how can I help you?'

'Ah, that's great, mate: I'm one of yer consular assistants here in Glasgow [I pronounce it Glass-Gow, not Glaz-Go] and yah see, you've probably heard about our Kylie being in the city today and doing a gig tonight?'

My voice rises in stress at the end of the sentence as I've learned from watching *Neighbours*. I go on: 'See, her old man has a bad history of heart problems, yer cardiology and all that, and well, she's raised loads of cash for the Australian Cardiology Society and well, here's the deal mate, she'd love to pop up and have a look around yer department and all that and maybe help raise some money for the heart people here: is that something you guys might be interested in?'

I do the upward inflection bit again, maybe a bit too good at that. Danvers answers: 'Well… Mr Ritchie – that's right, isn't it?'

'Yeah mate, Lance Ritchie at yer service.'

'Em, that sounds very interesting, Mr Ritchie, we'd love to see her.'

His voice is excited. Uh-oh. And then I push too far:

'Triffic, mate. Now listen, why don't you come on down if ye can to yer Nelson Mandela Place and we can sort out the details, how does that sound? Are you free right now?'

'I'm sure I can be.'

'Great! Well, let's see you in fifteen minutes, yeah?'

All the while I'm suspicious he has rumbled that it's me. So I go to the next level: 'Listen, ehm, are you and yer wife – ah, sorry mate, I'm presuming: you are married, right?'

'I am indeed.'

'Yeah, great. Marriage is a great thing. Well, how would you and yer wife like to join Kylie and the team for some tucker tonight? Yer not doing anything special tonight, are ya?'

Tucker: did I really say tucker? And Danvers answers: 'Tonight? No, not really, no.'

'Ah, that's swell, mate: come and join us after the gig, free tickets for that too!'

The phrase I've used is now shouting loudly in my head: *you're not doing anything special tonight?*

And then him answering: *not really, no.* Not really, no, I'm only supposed to be going round to one of my best friends' for dinner. He and his wife won't mind. Won't mind being stood up by Kylie Minogue. Bastard.

'Right then, ah'll see ya down at yer Nelson Mandela Street in fifteen, take care, mate!'

And then I put the phone down. What a swine. He knows we are cooking for them tonight, he knows we must have bought the food in by now. I pick up my coffee cup thinking that Danvers will be down to see me in a few minutes laughing his head off. But no, he doesn't show. The cardiology ward is directly above us and there is no sign of him. I look out the window at another dull grey day over Castle Street and to my horror see him walking briskly towards Strathclyde University and the centre of town. He's heading to Nelson Mandela Square! Shit.

There is no Australian consulate on Nelson Mandela Square. I rush out the coffee room and take the stairs three at a time and dash out the hospital, run across Castle Street without looking, and bolt town-wards, where I eventually catch up with him. I shout in Strine before reaching him: 'Danvers! DANVERS! Listen: *I'm* Lance Ritchie.'

He laughs, incredulous that he has been taken in, but... but it isn't that funny. Not really. I've overstepped a line. Laugh *with* people, not at them. There is a nasty taste in my mouth that has the dank flavour of mockery. And he knows it isn't that funny either – after all, he was going to disappoint us and dump our dinner together.

We eat that night anyway and our wives laugh at the story, but they too sense that all is not right. Danvers is forgiving and he will remind me of the story many times, partly in self-admonition, part self-mockery: how could I be so stupid? But also I'm sure he tells it as a way of reminding me that our friendship, like all friendships, has a limit: friendship does not permit thoughtless minor cruelties.

June 2016 and I'm at the Olympic Stadium in Berlin. I'm looking at Bruce Springsteen's face. The real Bruce: not a fake, not a fantasy. A friend who works on *Der Tagesspiegel* has blagged me a ticket. I've got none of Bruce's albums but I know the hits, I've heard how good he's meant to be live, and so I'm game. Springsteen's giant mug is projected onto a screen the size of a tennis court and I watch him grimace in furious concentration as he pulls off another histrionic guitar solo. He punches the air like a boxing champ, dances with some girls, gets a kid to come onstage and sing along with him. I watch as he paces along the front of a massive crowd and see that famous face break into several different variants of grin as he beams out to the many, many faces watching. His eyes want to lock with each fan individually and make them feel that extra bit special, a look that says: 'I know, I know: you *love* me.' Bruce winks and points and nods conspiratorially at them as if to say: 'Ah gotcha!' This is why he is loved. And suddenly he reminds me of someone.

Suddenly my mind is not seeing the face of a rock 'n' roll super-star any more; my mind is back in 1986. I'm seeing the face of a doctor called Ross McKenzie. My head is no longer in Germany: my head is back in Scotland again.

In Stirling, to be precise. JBF has told me that I have to rotate up in Stirling. One of the four consultants there is a laconic, dour chest specialist with a mordant sense of humour who acts as a medic at, ahem, boxing matches. He is unimpressed by arguments that say boxing is dangerous: he seems a tad indifferent to subdural haemorrhage. Says 'it's a risk'. And then there is McKenzie, mercurial Ross McKenzie. And it is McKenzie's facial expressions I recall when I watch Springsteen mugging for the masses.

On ward rounds McKenzie (Ross to his patients: 'Call me Ross') was in the habit of entering a bay of six patients where he would stand in the middle of the space, point at each patient, then beam widely at each of them, his eyes narrowing in glee. Then loudly, happily, he'd utter an expression like 'You OK?' or 'All right?' or 'You're doing great!' Just like Bruce.

After that he'd turn on his heels and head to the silence of the case note trolley in the corridor. The patients loved this performance. I don't think I ever saw him actually examine a patient once. At the trolley and out of earshot of the patients he would reveal a remarkable clinical perspicacity: he'd nod in the direction of one woman, now reading her *People's Friend*, smile again and say, sotto voce: 'She's got SLE, right?'

And he'd be spot on. Or, speaking of another woman: 'I think she's got MS.'

He would gurn at her too once she put down her magazine. Ross would flash his pearly whites in an attempt to cheer her up as she lay partly hemiplegic. He was an unfailingly curious man who handed me scientific papers on a daily basis. These had, however, a tendency to the obscure. There was something of the alchemist about him, always searching for some hidden secret knowledge that would unlock the door to some medical mystery.

He had a nose too for the occult forces in medicine: they threatened him; he saw ill will and conspiracy all around. He could sniff out the bad guys, the lackeys and yes-men who, he thought, ran the colleges and committees. This was the darkness of the profession and he represented the light: 'Watch out for the gatekeepers, JDQ. You know about the gatekeepers?'

I have a vision of guys in deerstalkers with the carcasses of dead grouse strung over their shoulders. I have no idea what he's on about. He expands: 'The gatekeepers, man! Oxbridge types that run the show. *The Friends*! Frivolous, non-entities, the lot of them.'

He must have noticed my sceptical look, or else sensed my mistaken vision of countryside bagmen. My silence provokes him: 'It's true! The gatekeepers are everywhere! Don't end up being one of the gatekeepers, JDQ. You know what happens in wartime, don't you?'

I frown in ignorance but play along: 'No, what happens in wartime?'

Now I have images in my head of a line of country gillies up against a wall about to be shot.

'They get rid of them! The gatekeepers are thrown out and we – you know, the government I mean – finally get the right man in place for the right job. That's what Churchill did, y'know, got rid of the gatekeepers and the call went out. The real talent was called in. So if you had a genius in Orkney or Wick or God knows where [why did I think at this point he might also mean Stirling?] Churchill would have him or her dragged down from the sticks and put in the place of some over-promoted nobody. But then after, when the war was over, ah well, the gatekeepers came right back. And they are still here today. Right now, JDQ, right now!'

Today you might imagine Ross as a proto-Dom Cummings figure on the lookout for talented weirdos. He'd go silent for a bit after this rant, open up some of his mail right there on the ward round, nod at a thin patient near the window and whisper: 'He's got lung cancer, am I right?'

And of course he was.

Later I learned that he would sneak into the ward early, look at the notes and examine the patients before we got there. He'd get the up-to-date information and then deliberately freak us out with his insights.

A week would pass without seeing him. I'd ask the other three consultants if they knew where Dr McKenzie was and they'd sigh. It was clear his absences were habitual. The chest physician was particularly scathing: 'Ross off playing with The Friends again?'

The Friends. Yes, he *did* go on about The Friends. Who they hell were The Friends?

I'd ask his secretary where he was: 'Damascus.'

'Right. I should have guessed.'

And then a month later: 'Montevideo.'

'Uh huh. Nice this time of year I'd imagine.'

And she would grin.

What in hell was he doing in Montevideo? All I knew about Montevideo was that there were guerrillas there called the Tupamaros. I'd learned that from a Scritti Politti song. I had a few Uruguayan stamps when I was a boy. They had pictures on them of odd trees with thick trunks called ombus. Ross was never to be found in places that were on the medical conference map: these trips of his were clearly not drug company jaunts to Lake Geneva or Chicago or Paris, no, no. He'd be checking out ombus, or maybe getting the gen on far-left terrorists for The Friends.

Another Monday, another day with his secretary: 'So, where's Ross this week?'

'Baku.'

'Of course! How could I forget?'

He's back. Dr McKenzie is back. I think about that name: Ross

McKenzie, yes, a perfect name for a spy. At last I've worked him out, all that jazz about gatekeepers and The Friends. I'll hint to him that *I know*. I'll say something that implies: *I get the picture*. And when later that day I do just that he just pulls his cheeky Springsteen grin, punches me gently in the shoulder, and whispers: 'I got ya!'

My inglorious research career continues, such as it is, squeezed into a busy clinical job as a registrar. A major boost comes from the arrival of Scott, the new senior registrar. I'd heard about him from Dr Hastie: 'Wears an earring. Bit of a rebel.'

Medicine doesn't dig rebels. Like that Chinese proverb about the nail that stands up: you are hammered back into place. Sartorially you are, if male, dressed in a cheap Marks & Spencer's suit, you wear lace-up black shoes, a white shirt, a clean white coat and a sensible tie. You look like TV's James Fox, their young BBC arts critic, who's forever saying: 'I think...' before appropriating the prior conclusions of older academics. Patter theft.

We dressed conservatively: there was a dress code and woe betide you if it was violated. Those late-twentieth-century Fridays when SHOs could wear comedy ties with pictures of Scooby-Doo were still a long way off in the future. Thankfully those days too are now long gone in the Benjaminian rubble of our collective past. I've never owned a comedy tie because I'm not a fuckin' comedian.

Women had to conform to flat shoes and unflattering dresses. No hint of cleavage, no hint of thigh. As a doctor you have to blend in, you must not draw attention to yourself; it's not about you. You must not appear sexualised; at work you are not a sexual object.

This was the 1980s, of course, and Scott – well, Scott was just ahead of the curve. In time the white coats would come off and wearing ties would be banned because of MRSA. Scott reads the *NME*. This is good. We quickly bond over a love of the Velvet Underground. Floridly imaginative, he might, I thought, be the irascible Lou Reed figure to my paranoid John Cale. Scott himself was sanguine about paranoia: 'Paranoia is when you *think* people are talking about you. I *know* people are taking about me, JDQ.'

He's right, they are. And with that he sticks his earring in place and heads down the well-worn stairs of the medical block at the Royal to bicycle home. He's ahead of the game; he knows exercise is good for you. But even bicycles were frowned upon back then. The following week JBF calls Scott into his office and tells him that the cycling look is unlikely to be consistent with a putative future consultant appointment.

Scott has a seriously impressive CV: he is a booster for clinical science and soon gets a study past the ethical committee where we can look at the effects of hypoglycaemia on, well... us. We were six 'normal' individuals – that is to say, we two plus four of our mates, other registrars. Here's the plan: we arrive at 5:30 a.m. (yup, 5:30 a.m.) and set out and label carefully the bottles we will fill with our blood samples. At six on the dot the subject (me today) is lying on a couch and has been cannulated. The insulin has been drawn up and is now injected into my arm veins. Nothing happens.

We talk about the gentle beauty of the Velvets' third album, reminisce over Scott's time working at a record shop in town, where he took delight in playing 'Frankie Teardrop' by Suicide very loudly. *Let's hear it for Frankie!* Some years later we read that Nick Hornby hates the song, if you can call it a song. 'Frankie Teardrop' is a violent American *cri de coeur*. Can't imagine our consultant bosses being big fans of Suicide. Physicians as a species, as good and proper paid-up members of the bourgeoisie, generally favour opera over neurotic New York City electronic proto-punk.

Twenty minutes pass: it's twenty past six in the morning now and I begin to feel quite odd. The fight-or-flight reaction kicks in. My adrenal glands are pouring out adrenaline in the face of my falling blood sugar. I'm beginning to sweat and wipe my brow. A minute later and I'm sweating buckets. Scott takes some blood from my cannula. Fills the bottles. He's also asking me questions from a sheet; some I find hard to answer despite their simplicity. Subtract nine from a hundred. I'm finding it hard to think straight, to rationalise, to concentrate. *Keep subtracting.* Eh? Ninety-one, eighty-two, seventy-three, sixty-four... forty-something. My blood sugar is very low now and I feel quite sleepy. Scott injects me with some glucose before I enter into a coma. I knew there were very good reasons for the deep questioning Scott had received earlier from the ethical team after he submitted plans for the study. My brain quickly soaks up the glucose and I feel better, but I'm not allowed to eat, not just yet. The study goes on, more samples, more questioning.

It is said that young men think about sex every fifteen seconds or so. I'm here to tell you that during profound hypoglycaemia you do *not* think about sex. You do not think about anything apart from... food. I lay there on the couch as Scott buzzed about filling the blood bottles and occasionally asking me what I made of Lou's *Metal Machine Music* or some such and all I could think about was what I planned to eat as soon as the study ended at eight-thirty. I would then have half an hour before the ward round started – that is to say, my normal day's work. I fully intended to gorge myself beforehand. I lay there woozy and thought about what I would eat.

Start with some breakfast cereal, yes, some Frosties maybe, those flakes, those sugar-coated flakes advertised by that trashy Tony the tiger, *grrrreat*, but... I'm feeling really odd now. Wonky thinking about tigers and tiger feet and that's right, that's right, that's right, that's right, I really love your tiger… Frosties, yes Frosties… I need Frosties NOW. Then after a bowl or two I might continue scoffing with maybe a big fry-up to follow, some sausages, bacon, mushrooms, maybe even some baked beans, yes, why not some sweet baked beans, Heinz beans, beanz meanz Heinz, cans of Heinz beans, or a can of Campbell's soup, Andy Warhol, Warhol, Warhol and the Velvets, Lou and John and the Exploding Plastic (*the exploding plastic what?*), then a voice asks me, Scott's voice once more: 'What is ninety-one minus nine?'

Ye whit? What was that? Scott is grilling me again: questions to see how my frontal cortex is dealing with hypoglycaemia, and all I can think about is how I'll wash that lot down with a cup of sugary tea and maybe get a Mars bar, a Mars Bar, a Mars a day helps you work, rest and play and maybe a Bounty bar too, yeah, why not? A taste of paradise. But I've no thoughts of sex on the beach under the coconut trees because I'm deeply, very deeply, hypoglycaemic.

The samples were duly analysed. Scott in turn wrote up the studies showing the effects of hypoglycaemia in normal subjects on other hormones, on various blood factors involved in clotting, on cerebral function. These were published in high-quality journals and Scott made sure I got my name on some of these. And I now knew what serious hypoglycaemia felt like: I now had an invaluable insight into what faced many people with Type 1 diabetes daily, sometimes hourly. This understanding will prove crucial for my future practice. Scott got me up and running as an endocrinologist.

9

FAILURE TO INDUCE HYPOGLYCAEMIA IN GLASWEGIAN ALCOHOLICS

Scott's face is sullen when we meet a few months later. He doesn't want to hear my ravings about the new 808 State or A Certain Ratio recording. 'They sound like Shakatak,' he murmurs scornfully. I want to defend the Mancunians but Scott interrupts. Dr Hastie has badgered him into taking on another study, one that Scott has no hopes for. The idea:

(a) We know that hypoglycaemia makes some people with diabetes become aggressive. We see this occasionally in those who have Type 1 diabetes. I should quickly point out that this was not my *personal* experience of hypoglycaemia. I was even more lethargic than usual during my time on the couch. Violence? No thanks, I'd rather have food please. *Food now!*

(b) Alcohol can be a contributory factor in the development of hypoglycaemia.

(c) Some alcoholics, non-diabetic alcoholics, can present to A+E with hypoglycaemia.

So Dr Hastie's hypothesis is simple: might hypoglycaemia be the cause of aggression in some alcoholics? Good question. How to test this? Scott has been given the task. Scott needs help.

And so we find ourselves in a psychiatric hospital near Celtic Park football stadium: 'Paradise' to fans of Glasgow Celtic. But we are very much this side of paradise: the wrong side. We are in the ECT room, a spartan, windowless place with a couch and two chairs for furniture. The dread equipment for applying electroconvulsive therapy to the terminally depressed sits on a tray. We are in this room armed with our blood bottles, our cannulation equipment and our syringes of glucose all drawn up. Fifty per cent concentrate of glucose in the form of dextrose is like syrup. Drawing this stuff into a syringe is like taking a can of Tate and Lyle's best and sucking it up, all thick and glutinous: it takes some effort to pull the syringe back and once full you notice a deep indentation in your thumb.

We are here in the ECT room with the patients who have been admitted for detoxification. All have agreed to the study; they have met with their psychiatrist first. The psychiatrists have explained what will happen to them. We go over it a second time. They have been formally assessed to have capacity. They know they will be bled. They know that the ethical committee has approved the study. And they can see the bottles of whisky that we have in a box under the couch. They are to be allowed one last drink. No one has said anything about violence. Scott and I are unarmed.

I ask myself now, older, more cautious: how on earth did the ethical committee ever pass this?

We crack open the bottles of whisky (blended, no expensive malts thank you very much) and give the men a generous tumbler each from a measuring jug. They grab the glass with trembling hands.

And then we wait and watch to see if they will go hypoglycaemic: we wait to see if they will turn violent on us.

So, just to be clear, we find ourselves secluded of a morning near Paradise, a place well known for hosting sectarian Saturday episodes of ultra-violence. Such demented affairs might feature nifty knife work, a riot of razor slashes, the occasional thunk of crossbow bolt on skull, the swoosh of a broadsword. Scott and I, then: ensconced with potential psychotics about to fuel up on copious amounts of booze. We dose… what might be the collective noun for jakeys?… a Fitzgerald of alcoholics some whisky to see if they'll go mental, to see if they will attack us.

None of them do. Scott's early scepticism about the study is well founded. This is that most frustrating of research experiences: a negative study. No one is interested in a negative study. But Scott is persistent; he writes it up and submits the results to several journals.

And gets it accepted, again with my name as a contributor. The title of the paper is a truism: 'Failure to induce reactive hypoglycaemia by drinking whisky and a mixer in Glaswegian alcoholic patients'.

Another month, another morning with Scott and the *NME*. He interrupts my gibbering about Haircut 100 and my admiration for their Arran sweaters to mention another study he has in mind. He's been talking to some surgeons. Oh no…

He says, given that:

(a) People with diabetes can develop neuropathy (damage to the nerves) as a long-term complication;

(b) These nerves can affect the gut, causing vomiting and diarrhoea: so-called autonomic neuropathy; and

(c) The anus is supplied by nerves.

Uh-oh. I know where this is going. He concludes with:

(d) The surgeons have developed a probe that can tell if anal func-
     tion is problematic and we could…

Probe. That's all I hear… *probe*. He's going to suggest that we stick
a probe up the arse of our patients. No. No, no, no. And again no.

'So, I've approached the ethical committee and they say we can
do it… What do you say, JDQ?'

'No.'

Scott is rightly dismissive of my squeamishness; he's seen that I'm
not cut out to be a real scientist.

'This is clinical *science*, man! C'mon! This one will be a positive
study, I'm sure of it. This will be worthwhile. And it'll be another
line on your CV.'

Another line on your CV. Maybe that's what physicians should have
carved on their tombstones: *This is the last line on my CV*. I've known
physicians who would adjust their CV on a daily basis. Tighten it up
to earn what used to be called 'discretionary points', a salary bonus.
But there are only so many times you can revise your CV before acute
catatonia is precipitated. I've narrowly avoided admission under the
psychiatrists after re-re-re-re-reading my CV before applying for a job.

Medicine as a career can be profoundly infantalist, with CVs a list of
achievements trying to scream: *Look at me, please look at me, pick me,
pleeeease!* Registrar Martin (*hi team!*) told us that we needed at least
thirty papers on our CV before going for senior registrar jobs and at
least fifty before getting a consultant appointment. This is an exagger-
ation these days; it probably was back then too, another way to wind
up the troops. 'First author, I mean,' Martin added, just to rub it in.

Scott does the probe study and it gets published. Anal function *is* impaired in some of our patients with diabetes: my hesitations were misplaced. This was an important piece of work.

Martin Hi Team! is a regular at Paradise. He isn't interested in Orange Juice or the Velvet Underground. Martin is interested in football. He's a Celtic fan: one of 'the bhoys'. When lecturing he is aware of the golden rule that everyone goes to sleep after six minutes and so he slips in another slide of the Lisbon Lions, winners of the 1967 European Cup. He approves of my Charlie Nicholas hairstyle. Martin sports a more coiffured affair, a Barry Manilow.

I'm at a conference in Denmark some years later presenting some data when I bump into Martin at the Tivoli Gardens. He asks me: 'What's with this little mermaid shit?'

Conferences are not my idea of fun. Diabetes is a global disease, a global threat; the pharmaceutical companies make a great deal of money out of the condition. One of the first things you encounter at an international medical conference on diabetes are the stands manned by the drones of the drug industry. These mini-marquees have become increasingly garish in design over the years. The language used by Big Pharma is sometimes demeaning and cheapened. The banners scream 'Reach the dream' and other such platitudes. But, hey, credit where credit is due, it looks like they might come to the rescue with viable vaccinations against Covid-19.

But some physicians behave badly at these meetings, shoulders hunched over with their tote bags laden with freebies. You hear boasts that they haven't spent a penny since arriving in San Francisco or Los Angeles.

And then at the conference itself egos are well and truly on parade. The Americans seem to shine brightest at this egregious display of self-promotion. It's all money and a bit of advertising to quite a few of them, I guess. At the end of their presentations they flash up a slide of their family, whom they will then proceed to thank at length. They dance their bright red laser pointer over some domestic scene. *I couldn't have achieved all this without my beautiful wife Tina and my lovely kids Tiger and Topher, and that's our golden retriever, Ike.*

Physicians are not always at their most generous at conferences. One popular spectator sport was the sight of a senior professor attacking some lowly registrar. This would be at question time following the registrar's presentation. These were not gratifying to witness. Thankfully I was not on the receiving end of such a vicious assault, but I do remember this minor humiliation: on stage in a room of about 1,000 people, I was asked if knew the molar concentration of IGF-1 that we had used when giving Bobby an injection. My look of incomprehension must have been something to behold. Molar? Isn't that something in your mouth?

Another time (again in front of hundreds of people) a senior asked if I could recall a line from *Hamlet* – something vaguely diabetes-related, to do with sugar and pious action and the devil. The crowd in front of me tiered as with the Globe theatre. Me as baby bear being baited.

Early autumn 2016 and I'm in the graveyard of St Peter and St Paul's Church in Aldeburgh, Suffolk, looking for the gravestone of Elizabeth Garrett Anderson, the first woman to qualify as a doctor in Britain. I can't find her tomb, but not far from the last resting places of Benjamin Britten and Peter Pears I stumble on a stone that says this:

DAVID PYKE

PHYSICIAN

Pyke! It was Pyke who grilled me about *Hamlet*. Pyke was legendary.

He would stand up from the audience, like a missile about to fire from a hidden silo, and announce imperially: 'Pyke, King's College' and then ask a forensic question. This might commend or condemn the speaker. His reputation as a physician was stellar. His gravestone said all it needed to say. He was a physician. At one time in my specialty he was *the* physician.

Standing amidst the orange- and lemon-coloured leaves contemplating his exit, I wondered if he might have been reassured that, now older, I can recall a few more lines of Shakespeare. There's that one from *Macbeth* about 'the way to dusty death'. Or was that from another Alistair MacLean book?

Staying with conference experiences, Danvers tells me he was once upbraided for his Glasgow accent at a national lecture he gave in London. He came away with the perfect rejoinder: 'I can do it again with subtitles for the hard of thinking.'

Danvers has another great, if horrible, story about deafness. A male nurse was sitting in with him at a clinic. A deaf patient comes into the consulting room for review but there's no interpreter. 'No problem,' says the nurse. 'I know how to communicate with the deaf.' Danvers is relieved. The nurse listens to Danvers introduce himself to the deaf patient by asking: 'How are you feeling?'

The nurse does not sign. The nurse does not know sign language. What's going on? The nurse then stares at the deaf patient and then impersonates what he *thinks* a deaf person might speak like. The nurse contorts his face and mouth and then slowly translates Danvers's question into something that sounds like the voice of that old deaf Labour MP Jack Ashley: '*Howsh... ahr... djew... feeleen?*'

Danvers had to kick the nurse out of his consulting room.

Glaswegian humour is gallows humour. A terminal laughter in the dark that is frequently disrespectful. Brueghel peasant humour:

insolent and distasteful, often boneheaded. Glaswegians, like Liverpudlians, think they are natural comics. Think they are a city of fuckin' comedians. Think they can make jokes about anything, even the Holocaust. This has something to do with the success of several talented comics born there but does not imply that all Glaswegians are funny, contrary to what many of us believe.

My dad knew a Holocaust 'joke'. He heard it in the crowd at a Scotland vs. West Germany game in the 1970s and we agreed the 'gag' confirmed man was irredeemable. This reminds me of a guy who volunteered for another of our studies. I had to sit and talk to him for hours and after the first five minutes it became apparent that he was no Adorno. He wasn't the sort to fret about the worthiness of poetry in a postlapsarian world. He was reading a book about the Second World War and I suppose I was impressed that he was reading anything given the reductive nature of his conversation. I asked if he liked reading books. He did and added, his face gurning: 'I love books about Auschwitz.'

Love. That was the word he used.

Glaswegian misanthropy is nothing if not balanced. I gave a copy of an A–Z book on Glasgow expressions called *The Patter* to a Palestinian doctor to help with his struggles understanding the locals. Two days later he threw it back at me.

Angrily he goes: 'Look under "A"!'

I skip to the page he has marked and find: 'Arab: as in "ya manky Arab"'. That's manky as in 'dirty'. I dumbly try to appeal to his sense of balance by asking had he looked up the entries for Catholics or Protestants or Highlanders or, God help us, the English. He's unimpressed.

When I later worked in England, the mere mention of Glasgow, or the sound of my accent, equated with incipient violence in some minds. This may not have been entirely unfair. I have never personally been in a fight, but I have come close.

A Christmas night out with the ward team at some corporate hotel on Cambridge Street. We are all mingling at the bar. There are a lot of people here and it becomes apparent that the hotel has booked at least three concurrent groups. I'm told one of them is the Govan police. I'm trying to get an order in. Professor JBF is here, standing about ten yards away, deep in conversation with Kris. I'm with my wife, waving a tenner in my hand in order to attract the barman's attention. A large man edges in through the crowd and stands beside my wife, pinches the silk of the dress on her arm and says: 'Nice material.'

My brain connects with my mouth without conscious thought of what might happen next: 'Fuck off.'

He stares at me with malevolent intent. I look around. The prof. is still in deep conversation with Kris and a few more of my colleagues have joined the group. I can't ask them to help me. What could I say?

'Hey guys, can you help get this thug to back off?'

Asking a Professor of Medicine in his mid-fifties to help you in a fight: it's not really an option. This is not something you would want to add to your CV. The goon orders: 'Outside!'

The Neanderthal has challenged me; he has called me out for a duel. *Outside*. I'm five foot seven; this isn't good. I avoid looking at my wife because I know she is scared and I don't want her to see that I'm pretty frightened too. I tell him we were just leaving anyway and we ease our way out of the crowd at the bar, past the prof. and Kris, still blissfully ignorant that their youngest registrar is about to be grievously assaulted. As the revolving doors beckon, I turn and see the thug is still following us with two of his equally tall and well-built friends. So I'm to fight three guys, each about twice my size. Great. We tumble through the doors and quickly jump into a waiting cab and tell the driver to push off fast, anywhere, do it now! The driver is quick: he accelerates and I look backwards and see the three guys chase the cab for a few seconds and then sit back and heave a sigh of relief. My pulse is rattling. I'm sweating. We can't sleep when we get home.

Next day I arrive at the hospital early and sip coffee in our office and wait for everyone to turn up. I can't concentrate on the newspaper or the copies of the *BMJ* that lie scattered around the table with its ring stains, twisted staples and rolls of micropore tape. Scott arrives: 'Well, that was some night!'

I'm assuming our precipitant departure is the talk of the town: 'Yeah, well…'

'I mean a good punch-up. That's not how you think a night out with the prof. is going to end up.'

'A fight?'

'Oh, yeah: I was looking for you after it happened. Didn't you see it?'

'No. I had to, uhm, leave early.'

'Well, you missed yourself. Some gynaecologist took on Frank. You know Frank the charge nurse. Argument over some girl, I think. Both of them slugging it out on the dance floor. You should have seen it!'

Later I learned that the three guys chasing my wife and I were from the Govan police.

I've just finished Paul Kalanithi's memoir of life as a neurosurgeon, *When Breath Becomes Air*. There is much to admire about this brave man and the book he left us after his sad and all too early death from lung cancer. In particular it is good for me to read that, after taking an MA in English literature, he felt that he 'didn't quite fit in an English department'. A possible career as an academic specialising in Walt Whitman was not for him. Life as a literary academic was never something I considered either, but as an outside interest I became almost dangerously obsessed with the life and work of Vladimir Nabokov. When I read Kalanithi's realisation that the academic life was not for him I recalled my first meeting with Pavel Dominik at a Nabokov conference in Nice.

Pavel mocked the pedantry and one-upmanship as the Nabokovian experts sweated over minutiae. We bonded laughing at some of the more extreme examples. Many would have pleased the great man himself; there were a few Kinbote-like figures in the room. *The European*, a now-defunct newspaper, interviewed us all. I later read with acute embarrassment that I was here in Nice talking about Nabokov, taking a break from doctoring, because it was 'better than gardening'.

I nod in tired recognition at Kalanithi's description of a typical lunch for a doctor: 'a Diet Coke and an ice-cream sandwich'. For me, in between clinics, a bag of Walker's crisps and a bottle of cherry-flavoured Volvic saw me through. Kalanithi's parents sound somewhat pushy. His father, also a doctor (a driven cardiologist), said to him: 'Find the guy who is number one, and score one point higher than he does'. Kalanithi strives for 'a nice catamaran', but he would never see it.

Perhaps it was my father (a bored taxman) who helped me to set my own goals just that little bit lower. In the great Pontoon game of life I'd learned from him to aim at eighteen and not twenty-one. If you go for twenty-one you end up bust. One day, when we were in our late teens and early twenties, Dad said to the four of us kids: 'You know, you guys are great but there's one thing you don't really have.'

We look at one another and then one of us asks: 'What's that?'

And he looks up and says: 'Talent.'

I laughed then frowned. He explains. We are all clever, all have good memories, and we are even, he concedes, quite bright. But we have no real talent. We cannot play any musical instruments. We cannot sing or perform. We can't paint or write poetry. Most of all, he notes: 'Look, let's face it: none of you is likely to be the new Mozart.'

So that's what we are up against. Mozart. Forget pushy Indian uncool cardiology fathers like poor Kalanithi's, using passive-aggressive techniques to inspire their sons and daughters onto the heights of medical academia. Our father wanted us to be the new Mozart.

At one point in his US training Kalanithi is told by the chief resident: 'Neurosurgical residents aren't just the best surgeons – we're the best *doctors* in the hospital.' This makes me laugh out loud. Any hospital physician in the UK will tell you that a phone call with the equivalent grade here, the neurosurgical registrar, goes something like this:

'Switchboard, can you get me the neurosurgical registrar, please.'

While they are bleeping you rehearse the story in your mind. A young man has come in with a sudden onset headache, the worst he's ever had in his life, he describes it as if he has been hit on the back of his neck with a hammer, a history so clear-cut for a subarachnoid haemorrhage that he could have read it from a textbook. You're worried about him. He's young. People die from these intra-cerebral bleeds. You've scanned him. There's blood in his brain. He needs to be transferred to the neurosurgeons. The phone crackles into life: 'Yuh?'

That's how the neurosurgical registrar addresses his fellow professional. *Yuh?*

You tell the story. And then he says: 'Do an LP.'

He wants you to do a lumbar puncture, but it is clear from the scan, it is clear from the consultant neuroradiologist's report that there is blood in there. You do not need to do an LP to confirm this and you tell him so. His reply?

'Do an LP.'

The duel is on: 'Look, as I've said, the neuroradiologist has said the findings are in keeping with a subarachnoid bleed. Please take this man. He is inappropriately managed here.'

'Do an LP.'

'Listen, if you do not agree to take this patient, I will phone your boss.'

'OK. Send him to our ward please.'

Each and every day a physician in Britain has an obstructive, rude and downright unpleasant conversation with a near-aphasic neuro-surgical registrar; it has been this way for more than twenty years. Best doctors in the hospital? Many would argue the most impolite.

Of course every specialty thinks that they are the best in the hospital, the best in the world. Cardiologists think this because the pump is all-important: if the heart packs up then it's game over. Renal physicians think they are the only doctors who understand the body's fluid balance, the sodium and potassium shifts. Neurologists think they're the smartest because they know about the brain. But of course it is the diabetologists/endocrinologists who are truly the last of the old-style general physicians, because they need to be cognisant of brain, cardiac, renal, liver, gut *and* sexual function, because when you get down to it *everything* is endocrinology, everything is mediated by chemical messengers, hormones. So, apologies to Dr Kalanithi. Endocrinologists are the best doctors in the hospital. He's up there in literary medicine's Valhalla shaking his head muttering: *Yeah, right. Whatever, Quinnie.*

Kalanithi talks brilliantly about WICOS: Who is the captain

of the ship? He means the American practice whereby many specialties chip in with a patient but no one seems to be in overall charge. Neurologists are particularly guilty of doing this. They see a ward patient on request and then write a suggested plan in the notes and say bye-bye. These suggestions might include a smart-arse request such as 'do Yo antibodies'. Yo antibodies: what the fuck are they? Antibodies to hip-hop? Antibodies to Public Enemy? The neurologists write these instructions and never deign to visit the patient again. The captain of the ship needs to be a general physician. And quite often that would mean an endocrinologist. But the real question is: why has this American WICOS problem arisen in the first place?

Private medicine has something to do with this. Stick to your own niche. Count the money. Don't get involved in complex cases. Don't try to be a Master Mariner.

Poor Kalanithi. His own illness is fearlessly described, as are his brutal treatments with chemotherapy. He died way too young. He would have gone on to write many more fine books if he had lived. His final message would appear to be this: be merciful. He's right. I should be more merciful when talking of neurosurgeons. After all, one day I may need one.

Kalanithi sits on one shoulder, angel-like, pleading for mercy. On the other, the devil: Dr Louis-Ferdinand Céline, arguing: 'These literary men are the limit... so afflicted with me-me-ism... And what about doctors? Just as bad!'

Being merciful can be very hard in this vale of tears where others do not play by your rules, *the* rules, or any concept of the word 'rules'. There are devils out there – like terrorists, for instance. Let's hear from them.

10

ENTER THE IRA AND THE KID
CREOLE OF HORMONES

How the IRA changed my life. An intervention by the Irish Republican Army led me to finally leave my country and head for London just as JBF had predicted. The Provisional IRA to be exact.

As the '90s began, a consultant job in Glasgow was advertised and Cycling Scott was the favourite to get the post. And if he got that job then his place on the SR rotation would be vacated. I was now one of the next in line. But then JBF phones and asks me to head to his office: 'Did you see the news last night?'

'About BSE? John Gummer eating a hamburger?'

The rare killer disease bovine spongiform encephalopathy was then much in the news, ditto said politician. Happier times! JBF gets back on point: 'No, about Northern Ireland.'

'Can't say I did. Another shooting?'

'No, not this time. The IRA kidnapped a woman and they threatened to kill her. She's married to a Tory, well, a man who has set himself up as a prospective Conservative candidate. A Conservative candidate in Northern Ireland. Think about that.'

'Right.'

Ian Gow, a Tory MP, had recently been killed by a car bomb near Pevensey in East Sussex. JBF is staring at me patiently as if I'm meant to get the punchline. I'm thinking ... *and*? Why is JBF talking to me about an IRA kidnapping? He's up to speed on haemopneumothoraxes, but what's all this about the IRA?

'Well, anyway, she got away somehow but I've been having some conversations with people. Turns out her husband is none other than Neil Steele. You know him, right?'

'No, I don't. Should I?'

'Yes, well, you see, JDQ, he's a consultant diabetologist in Belfast and he needs to get out of town ASAP. Clearly.'

'Clearly.'

'And you know what this means, don't you?'

This means that the job application I'd put in to Bart's in London for a laugh should now *not* be withdrawn. Why? Because this move by the IRA would mean that Scott would *not* get the job in Glasgow; that job would go to Neil Steele. And I would have to wait, JBF was hinting strongly, for some years to get an SR post in my own country. All because of an IRA threat.

Bart's shortlist me and I train it down to the capital. I'm to meet the head honcho there and I knock on his office door. He greets me, asks me to sit down, and I note immediately the magnificent view he has of St Paul's. Wren's dome intensifies my sense of intimidation. This is a serious place. He asks me what I would like to do if I got the job and I blandly list off the weekly timetable as a warm-up. I say something like: 'I'm looking forward to doing the pituitary clinic on a Wednesday,' when he raises a hand. He's riled: 'Stop. The pituitary clinic isn't on a Wednesday. Who told you that?'

His manner is suspicious, superior. I'm placatory, careful; I sense this is a man used to subservience. 'Well, it said Wednesday on the job plan.'

'Show me!'

I hand the pages over to him and then he suddenly grabs his desk phone with his right hand while his left stretches to the skies in frustration. He starts blaring: 'This young man here has come all the way down from Glasgow and you've sent him the WRONG job description, do you hear me? The WRONG job!'

And at this point his other raised hand slams down on the table with a very loud bang. I'm not sure I want to work with this guy, even if he is one of the best endocrinologists in the country.

A few weeks later I hear I've been shortlisted again, this time for King's, and I get the job. We're moving to London! Neil Steele, the Ulster Tory, got a job somewhere else in Scotland and Cycling Scott was duly appointed to Glasgow as a consultant but there was still no talk of a local SR job that I could have gone for. This is how it works. This is how lives are changed.

Amanda is another registrar in Glasgow on the team, a younger trainee diabetologist, who is now tasked with arranging my leaving do. We are in a Greek restaurant on the trendier west side of the city. Maybe twenty of us around a table, colleagues and secretaries, as the hummus and falafel and olives arrive. Amanda is on my left. At the top of the table sits one of the older secretaries. She wears polka dot dresses with large bows on the back; an older New Romantic. The meal goes well. People are happy with their food; even the rough retsina gets a cheer. And then it is time for speeches and a presentation. I'm honest about how I'll miss the team and how much I've enjoyed working with them. Then I'm handed a large oblong wrapped package and it's clear that this is a painting or a print. Amanda speaks up: 'Danvers told us that you loved art and so we thought about buying you a picture.'

I express my heartfelt thanks, but I'm reluctant to open the package because I remember that incident with Danvers and Lance Ritchie and the Australian consulate: he's not forgotten that Kylie Minogue prank.

'Go on, open it!'

The secretary with the polka dots is insisting this from the top end of the table and I give in. As I'm ripping open the brown wrapping paper, I have a memory of being with Danvers at an art show in the Merchant City. We saw some abstract expressionist-influenced canvases by the fifth Beatle, Stuart Sutcliffe. Maybe they've bought one of those for me... surely not? Sutcliffe's paintings were a riot of scarlet and black streaks, potent images of angst, Pollock with a migraine. Sutcliffe's tragic early death from a brain haemorrhage seemed bizarrely preordained. His pessimistic canvases are like a dark portent.

I've got the wrapping off now and the print is open to view. The picture is not a Sutcliffe, but it is immediately clear that Danvers has assumed my taste in art tends to the traumatised. I'm looking at a vision of two naked figures clinging to one another as they descend into a dark pit of hell. Imagine a sub-Kokoschka rendering of pain: Vienna circa 1910. I should have told Danvers how much I love Matisse. A voice from the top of the table breaks the uneasy silence: 'You don't like it, do you?'

The polka dot secretary is onto me.

'It's... it's very interesting.'

'Yeah, but you don't like it, do you?'

She's perceptive; my face is almost certainly giving clues to my disappointment. The artist Ed Ruscha is well known for his comment about one's immediate response on looking at an artwork. He describes this as either a 'Wow, huh?' moment or, much better, a 'Huh, wow!' reaction. So what was the look on my face right now? I think this was being read as a 'Holy fuck.'

I try to speak: 'No, no. It's very interesting, it really is. It will grow on me. I'm sure.'

Yeah, grow like a fungus perhaps, like athlete's foot. No, worse – more like mucormycosis. Mucormycosis: a fungus that rips through your face, your head. A fungus you don't want to know. I vow to stash the picture at the back of the least accessible, most obscure part of my house. No, make that my parents' house. The meal goes on. Fifteen minutes later Polka Dot asks again: 'You don't like it, do you?'

I ignore her. I turn and talk to Amanda for a bit. Thank her again for buying me the present. She says: 'Danvers said you'd like it. He was sure it was your taste. Said something about an exhibition the pair of you checked out.'

Bloody Stuart Sutcliffe: this is all Stuart Sutcliffe's fault! Why did he have to die? Why did those slaughterhouse images become his legacy? Why didn't he end up at Shea Stadium playing bass, why wasn't he playing on *Sgt Pepper* rather than ending up as a tragic face peeping out from Peter Blake's cover? Another fifteen minutes pass. And then Polka Dot tries again. She's bugging me. Her voice is needling. She wants the truth: 'You *really* don't like it, do you?'

All right: she wants the truth. Right then, I'll give it to her: 'OK. Look… ah… it's not really my taste, but…'

What was my taste at that time? Odilon Redon's pastels at the Musée d'Orsay, Warhol's pop disasters, the Glasgow colourists. Why didn't they just get me a cheap poster, a Bunty Cadell view of Iona? But then I become aware of acute distress at my side. Amanda has stood up and now she's running out of the restaurant in tears and soon I'm chasing after her down Great Western Road and I'm shouting: 'AMANDA! I'm sorry Amanda, Amanda, I'm really sorry...'

I'd like to say this was the moment I realised one day I could become an art critic. But I can't. I was a jerk. There are limits to being absolutely truthful.

I met Amanda decades later, after I'd published some art criticism. She is a busy consultant and we talked about hormones and then that awful night. She laughs and says she has forgiven me when I apologise yet again for my bad behaviour. Amanda tells me that the secretary in the polka dot dress has just had surgery for cancer. The secretary had only been teasing me that evening. I hear Kalanithi's voice in my head: *Be merciful.* I hope she's OK.

Before leaving Glasgow, I worked a year on the academic unit with one Arthur Ferris. We called him AF, like the dysrhythmia called atrial fibrillation. Arthur was a gentle obese man with a waspish sting of a wit; he was not afraid to inflict this on any slacker. He too had a love of clinical signs and would take great joy at the bedside when he found delayed reflexes and the like. His voice was high-pitched and wheezing, his movements slow, but his enthusiasm for diagnosis was infectious. He'd say rapidly: 'Yes, yes, that's right' if you spotted a sign. *Yesyesthatsright.*

Arthur AF wore braces that hitched his trousers to somewhere around his umbilicus. Danvers called him the August Darnell of Endocrinology, the Kid Creole of Hormones. Arthur loved too the inconsistencies of medicine, of life itself. He would delight in pointing out a very thin lady walking away from his clinic room and ask if I could guess her thyroid-stimulating hormone (TSH) level. The normal range varies from lab to lab but typically falls between 0.4 and 4 milliunits per litre. Patients with an overactive thyroid (hyperthyroidism) usually lose weight and their TSH level is consequently low: the pituitary has turned down its stimulating effect on the thyroid. This is a classic example of the near-ubiquitous and beautifully logical form of endocrine system control: negative feedback. As a corollary, people with an underactive thyroid (hypothyroidism) gain weight and have a high level of TSH. Arthur watches the thin woman leave the clinic and says: 'So, see Olive Oyl over there? Guess what her TSH is...'

'Uhm, I think it might be undetectable. Under 0.03?'

'Wrong! Ha, ha! You'll be intrigued to know that in fact her TSH yesterday was ten. Yes, yes, that's right. *Ten*.'

And then maybe the following week he'd point out some Giant Haystacks waddling down a corridor and grill me again: 'What's that guy's TSH, then?'

'You're not going to get me this time, he must be hypothyroid, I'll say twelve.'

'Wrong again, JDQ! He's overactive! His TSH is undetectable! *Yesyesthatsright*.'

Real life is not like textbooks. Although he was slow moving, I recall a day when AF's mild manner splintered. A young lady with a pituitary tumour had fallen pregnant. The pituitary lies underneath the optic chiasm, a junction of nerves that connects the brain to each retina. Pituitary tumours can swell in pregnancy. Compression of the chiasm can cause blindness. I was highly impressed by the speed of his actions and his urgent referral to the neurosurgeons. (This time there was no Neanderthal *yuh?* on the phone. No *yuh?* to the August Darnell of endocrinology.) Her sight was saved.

Around this time we also cared for a middle-aged woman with a malignant adrenal gland tumour, and the rapidity of her decline was shocking. We tried some rarely used drugs, but to no avail. Her husband was a famous actor and I remember the other patients on the ward wanting his autograph even as he was mourning. He himself died a year or so later: dying on the vine in his grief.

Dealing with actors and actresses, as patients, can be an odd experience. Almost all I've known have been delightful in that way we associate with the classic luvvie clichés. Calling them into your clinic room can be disconcerting. You call them by their real name but soon confront a person that you know only by their TV personality and name, their soap star character. A decade maybe of knowing them as a crook or a serial killer or a philanderer and you have to talk to them as if all that is now forgotten; they are in real life someone else entirely, someone frail, ill and frightened.

Years later I get a call one evening from a trainee: 'Dr Quin, we thought we'd better phone you about a patient.'

'Aye. No problem. What's up?'

'It's an old lady in her eighties who we think had a stroke yesterday. She needs to come in because her daughter is having difficulty getting her mum out of bed, toileting and so on…'

An everyday admission then: what are they not telling me?

'Sounds OK to me. Sure, bring her in. Anything else?'

'Ah, yes. We think her daughter was, or is, a famous actress and so we thought it best to call you and let you know, just in case.'

They mean just in case the media get a hold of this private information. Leaks happen. Bystanders accepting a wad of notes from a journalist, stuff like that.

'Sure. What's the daughter's name?'

'Bastedo. A Miss Alexandra Bastedo.'

Alexandra Bastedo! Oh, boy. Suddenly I'm eleven again and at home with my parents watching *The Champions*, a TV show set in Geneva. The opening credits had Bastedo and two guys standing beside the famous fountain, the Jet d'Eau. All three had super-powers gifted to them by Tibetan shamans after they survived a plane crash. They use these powers to tackle crime and evil: hence their title, the Champions. Bastedo was the epitome of European chic and sophistication. She had chiselled Grace Kelly cheekbones, a Slavic facial geometry; she wore cream and sky-blue Chanel suits.

'See you in fifteen.'

Miss Bastedo is older, of course, but no less beautiful. She care-fully listens to my explication on her mother's illness, her prognosis, what we will do for her. All the while I'm looking at those TV eyes and know that she knows. She knows as a boy I was in a juvenile form of love with her.

There was another prof. in the academic unit, an expert on bone. He didn't seem to care much for any other organ. He had a six-bedded ward where he would admit patients with osteoporosis, an unthinkable option today. They would be admitted for four days. *Four!* There was an admissions protocol and each patient would have an investigation per day: bone density estimation, bloods taken and so on. On one of these days the patient would have a bone biopsy. This was a job for the registrar.

My sincere apologies to everyone who underwent a bone biopsy under my hand during that year. Here's what this involved: infil-tration of local anaesthetic over the iliac crest, where your hipbone flares, what many people call 'my side'. You'd wait a few minutes for the local to take effect. You tried to get the local delivered to the per-iosteum, the thin layer of tissue covering bone. Then you took out a small cookie-cutter thing, a steel tube with serrated edges that had a diameter of around half an inch. After a small incision with a scalpel through the skin you would place the cookie-cutter on the bone, on the patient's side, and press down firmly and rotate. *Ker-unch.*

As I write I can still feel the grinding twist as the cutter dug into bone. If the patient had osteoporosis the process was often very easy, the bone having a soft consistency, as if hacking into the icing of a large wedding cake. If the bone were tougher, that is to say normal, then it would feel like cutting into a piece of hard wood. Pulling the cookie-cutter out was not unlike a dental extraction. If the patient had one of the rarer forms of osteosclerosis (hardened bones) then the process might be compared to trying to biopsy a diamond. Impossible. You'd get the distinct impression that the teeth of the cutter were being ground down themselves.

The professor told me that it was essential that we performed these biopsies for research purposes, and I believed him and so, like a functionary of the Third Reich, I did as I was told. I carried them out. I can only plead pathetically *à la* Nuremberg that I was young and obeyed orders.

Remembering bone biopsies calls to mind an even more barbaric practice: bone marrow aspiration taken from the sternum. I think this is now more likely to be taken from the iliac crest (where we did those bone biopsies). Back in the early 1980s we would regularly perform sternal aspirates. Again we would put some local in and then crunch into the breastplate. There was a metal guard in case you pushed too hard. This was to prevent you going straight through the chest wall and into the aorta. I'm told this did happen in the twentieth century, albeit rarely.

We were also encouraged to do liver biopsies, though I managed to avoid these. Why? Well, this was before routine ultrasound guidance and I heard from seniors that sometimes reports on these came back from the histology lab saying things like 'normal kidney' or, worse because it is much more vascular, 'normal spleen'. Or, worst of all, 'normal liver, kidney, gut and spleen'. What some called a 'kebab' biopsy. Thankfully, modern imaging techniques have significantly reduced the incidence of such disasters.

My time in the academic unit was ending. Academics could be condescending about clinicians. They were rarely, if ever, on call more than once a month and that irritated me. Some struggled to see three patients in an afternoon's clinic session. A few couldn't communicate properly with ordinary people.

The problems of the NHS in Scotland were not new ones: it was time for me to see if things were any better down south. From the high land and hard rain to the green and pleasant. *Leave it aht.*

PART TWO

ENGLAND 1992–2016

11

TORTURE

London in the early 1990s. My new boss was an intense, taciturn man, an anti-racist Zimbabwean (a fact he was rightly proud of, refusing to countenance the word 'Rhodesian') who started work at 6 a.m. His secretary was the toughest gatekeeper I have ever met, but we seemed to get on.

Meetings were brisk, laser-focused and highly informed on the latest developments in endocrinology, as if there were an unspoken challenge to out-quote one another on the most recent papers. JBF had warned me to prepare several talks before leaving Scotland: he was correct; within days I was timetabled to perform. My fellow SR was Patrick, a real Londoner who helped me integrate with ease. He taught me the basics of blotting: the careful pipetting of fluid into gels, a technique that enabled us to quantify proteins. He was an inveterate smoker and would call multiple time-outs from our research bench sessions to light up in one of the car parks. He'd quiz me with the same intellectual ferocity as our boss: 'Tell me what you know about IGFBP-5.'

Which would be precisely f-all. BP stood for binding protein: this I knew. I was aware there were three binding proteins for IGF-1, named easily 1, 2 and 3, but 5? Was there a 5? Is he having me on? Is this a test? Patrick is quick to let me know that there are now thought to be six binding proteins.

Patrick was also anti-racist and hearing his enthusiasm for multi-cultural London was a marked change from the derogatory non-sense I'd heard for many years in Glasgow with reference to Arabs and people from the Indian subcontinent. He also had a deep love for jazz and Brixton nightlife. Soon, with his tips, my wife and I hit the town.

We went clubbing in subterranean vaults near London Bridge, the tunnels off Tooley Street. There was a brick-walled bar lined with shiny electric blue bottles of water: no spirits, just Evian water. I learned that the DJ was one of the Two Lone Swordsmen. This was their *nom de guerre*. Londoners, I was quickly reassured, did not carry swords; this was good. But they did have guns. Racist white taxi drivers in Brixton would warn us that some people *aroun' 'ere* carried shooters. Whatever. And, reassuringly, people my age (just over thirty) were at the club: this just didn't happen up in Glasgow. In Glasgow we'd have been told to head off home to bed, granddad.

And suddenly people that I didn't know, the beautiful people, were hugging us both. This *really* never happened in Glasgow. What was all this lovey-dovey stuff about? Ecstasy, of course. That explained the bottles of water.

We would stay out after midnight in bustling Soho at Bar Italia with its football posters or sip rose-flavoured vodkas in Kensington. Best of all were the nights at the Brixtonian bar, like something out of an Ian Fleming fantasy, with its outrageously stylish Jamaican couples swaying on the dancefloor to dub reggae. Other nights we'd cruise the city in our old Peugeot 205 listening to the pirate radio stations: the orange streetlights of Camberwell glinting in the pools of rainwater by the roadside. The manic voices would talk of posses; the music a clattering of electronic pads and woozy synthesisers with the DJ machine-gunning his patter: 'This one is going out to all my bros in Streatham.' We loved the band Renegade Soundwave – a betrayal of sorts; no one in Glasgow seemed to like them, what with their talk of gangland malarkey, shooters and robberies. We got into the Kray Twins' mythology and the Richardsons'. Embarrassing. We hung out at the Blind Beggar, the Pride of Spitalfields; drank pints of Fullers. And we would head up west too. Sneak into the Ivy at 5 p.m. when we were flush and you could get a table. Order Manhattans. Illegally park off Piccadilly Circus. Blow our money.

London meant improv comedy clubs, nights at the theatre, good flat warm ale outside pubs in the summer. *Outside!* After a lifetime of dark dives hiding from the rain we could now sup a pint bathed in sunlight. London meant galleries, museums. I would get to know the National and discover the beauty of the Van Eyck Arnolfini Portrait. And this too: there was something stirring from Goldsmiths Art School. Young artists were doing simple cheeky things with coloured dots on walls, making text paintings with the names of the famous.

A couple of years later and some of these artists were famous themselves. There was a crazily expensive restaurant decorated with photographs of a young woman eating a banana, another of a young man in a gorilla suit. There was a huge ashtray hung upside down on the ceiling and some medicine cabinets lining the walls. The writer Jonathan Meades disapprovingly called it 'self-conscious stunt art'. But something was happening, a scene that reminded me of Glasgow in 1980, artists and musicians helping one another. That restaurant, Quo Vadis, was, ironically, housed in a building where Marx used to live. It was a time of great music. The capital was on fire again. We walked around Clerkenwell, Tufnell Park, Chalk Farm and

Camden, then south to Peckham, Dulwich, Battersea and Clapham, soundtracked by Saint Etienne and Blur: *So Tough* and *Modern Life Is Rubbish*. The city was alive. London in 1993 was the place to be.

One of the other bosses at King's Hospital was an academic who appeared to be scared senseless by clinical work. He couldn't (or wouldn't) communicate with patients on any kind of straightforward level. He would use complicated jargon that even his students struggled to understand. I watched him face a young woman recovering slowly after a clot in her lungs. This had nearly killed her. Instead of reassuring her that she would live, he said: 'We will test you for Factor S and Factor 5 Leiden, OK?'

One Friday afternoon when he was supposed to be the consultant on call he phoned me: 'I'm really sorry, John, but I've totally forgotten about the rota! I'm afraid I'm now in Paris so could you possibly step up and cover me and, look, I'm afraid my phone is running low and, oh shit, the car is about to go into a tunn—'

I cover him. Two weeks later and it's a Saturday morning around 8 a.m. My phone rings and it's him again: 'Meet me in the café of the Ritz at ten. Bring your wife.'

His apology for Paris takes the form of a slap-up breakfast meal in the baroque dining room of the grand hotel. Ostentatiously wealthy guests chomp down on rashers of bacon, thick sausages, Stornoway black pudding and maybe a glass or two of Sekt.

Not all of my new colleagues in London were as cosmopolitan or as enthusiastic about London's glories. One physician was explicitly racist and made comments in front of several witnesses. I gleaned quickly that the majority distrusted him and yet I heard years later that he made professor somewhere. Probably learned how to 'finesse' his remarks.

Here's a word I learned: megalothymia. I think that was this prof's problem. It could even be said that this is *our* problem in Britain. Megalothymia: the need to be recognised as superior to others.

Those at the very top can seem distant from those on the front line. Maybe that's how they got there in the first place: by quickly escaping the carnage at the front door. Many years later, in the twenty-first century, I would note, in the light of the threat of five-day strikes by junior doctors, a statement from the Academy of the Royal Colleges. The Academy is meant to be the view of the collective, the presidents of all the colleges. The statement was short and said that the Academy was 'disappointed at the prospect of sustained industrial action by junior doctors'. There was no mention of disappointment at the government.

The junior doctors' strike of 2016 resulted in a short state of civil war in British medicine. One columnist at the *Telegraph* openly called junior doctors 'idiots'. The same paper that day had a report of a maternity unit in the (then recently deposed) previous Prime Minister's constituency closing because of a shortage of junior doctors. Conspicuously, it was the Patients Association that strongly urged the Department of Health to resume meaningful discussions with the junior doctors.

One of the most recent pronouncements from the chair of the Academy in 2020 (pre-Covid-19, of course) is that doctors can no longer 'sit on their hands', that they should stop moaning and blaming the government for the problems of the NHS. That hasn't aged well.

The Zimbabwean professor of medicine hears that there is a consultant job coming up in Brighton. We arrange to meet at 6 a.m. in his office. A large canvas by an Aboriginal artist lines his wall. 'Here's what I suspect they will ask you.'

He lists about six questions he thinks they are likely to pose. Says he thinks this is the job for me, shakes my hand and wishes me good luck. He makes sure that I leave at 0615 prompt. I doubt I've ever met a more industrious doctor.

A couple of weeks later I get the job. Brighton! I'd always wanted to work by the sea: those trips to Malta as a boy had left a deep influence on my life. Five years of university study and then another ten as a 'junior' doctor; now I'm a senior at last. I'm elated.

I was called back into the interview room after a nervous wait to be told I've got the post. I'm ecstatic that I have secured a long-term position by the seaside. Suddenly I hear a flapping sound that seems to be coming from somewhere south of my head, a flapping, yapping, noise that appears to be coming from... me. I look down and see that it's one of my shoes. I walk briskly across the car park to meet my wife waiting and see that the sole of one of my shoes has come loose. I look like some circus clown. I flap-flap-flap to our car and laugh in relief when she switches on the ignition. We take off immediately for Newhaven and the Dieppe ferry. I'll splash out on a pair of espadrilles in France, imagine I'm Jean-Paul Belmondo in *Pierrot le Fou*.

I'm on call for the first time in Brighton... and I'm at home. Consultants can do on call from home: hurrah! We're renting a flat on Lewes Crescent. Regency architecture; white as wedding cake. Nick Cave lives hereabouts now. I can discuss cases while looking out at the marina and the sea.

But such luxury is now in real doubt. How long will consultants be non-resident in the twenty-first century? Given the intensity of medicine these days and the shortage of junior doctors it seems inevitable that consultants will spend more time on-site. Many paediatricians at consultant level are already resident, ditto obstetricians. Covid-19 has already enforced this for many physicians.

11 p.m. on call and I phone up the registrar; he hasn't asked for help so far: 'How goes it?'

'Oh, not bad, busy, but we're in control.'

This is what registrars often say, something non-committal, almost reassuring, a hurried reply that really means: *Thanks for calling, boss, but let me get on with it.*

'So how many have you had in?'

'Maybe about twenty.'

I can hear in his voice that he wants to press on, needs to see someone else; I've been there. So I keep it brisk: 'Anything interesting?'

'Well… there was a guy in his forties earlier this afternoon with a good story for a subarachnoid, confirmed on the scan, so he's gone to the neurosurgeons.'

'Good. They've taken one without a lumbar puncture for once. Anything else?'

I can sense the urgency in the charged environment surrounding him; can hear the noise in A+E, the bleeps, phones a-ringing incessantly, annoyingly, as the midnight hour approaches: 'Yeah, there's an elderly gentleman with a stroke, again confirmed on the scan. Couple of chron brons.'

He means chronic bronchitics. The textbooks split these into pink puffers and blue bloaters. The thin pink-coloured ones gasp away, but we fear the cyanosed bloaters most; they can't recognise that their carbon dioxide levels are rising. When this happens they can slip into a coma that is often irreversible. He goes on: 'Few chest pains. Three pneumonias, all elderly, all stable. A DKA doing well on fluids.'

Diabetic ketoacidosis again: barely a day goes by in hospitals the world over without one patient being admitted with DKA. This is testament to the difficulty people have giving themselves insulin injections daily in order to live. You try jabbing yourself four times a day. Before dashing off the line he adds one more comment: 'Oh, and there's a young guy, twenty-three, he's been in for a week or so. HIV positive. He's got meningitis caused by one of those odd funguses. The team looking after him has said he's DNAR.'

Do not attempt resuscitation. This young man I'm hearing about is dying from AIDS and he is twenty-three years old. It is 1994.

I stare out at the night. This is the last patient the registrar mentions on his list. The patient is an afterthought: a 23-year-old afterthought. We cannot save a 23-year-old. I ask does he know if the poor lad is comfortable and I am told that he is. There is nothing I can do. He joins a now long list of young people who have died from AIDS.

I had never looked after any patients with HIV in Glasgow. There were a couple of junkies with the infection, but they were cared for in a hospital called Ruchill over in a rough, unloved part of town. They had an iron lung at Ruchill that I saw as a student. The metal coffin-shaped horror sat malevolently alone in an otherwise empty room. I did part of my psychiatric training at Ruchill and visited an ex-nun with anorexia hiding in one of the burnt-out estates. She was a spectral vision, a pallid Virgin Mary as painted by El Greco. There was only one car parked on the street outside, a scarlet Porsche owned by the local heroin dealer. What was she doing here?

Edinburgh had the *real* heroin problem back then, as documented in Irvine Welsh's *Trainspotting*: Glasgow junkies didn't seem to share their needles as much.

The newspapers called HIV and AIDS a 'gay plague'. The poisonous journalist John Junor infamously said: 'There's no poofs in Auchtermuchty.' Scotland wasn't exactly a beacon of tolerance back then. When Waterstones opened a gay section in its Ca' d'Oro shop near Central Station it had one shelf. There was a Burroughs, I think, and a couple of books by Edmund White. I remember this conversation from that time too: 'Did you hear about Arto?'

Three consultants working in the west side of the city talking about a colleague in his early forties: 'I hear he's... unwell.'

'He is indeed. They say he's dying.'

'Dying, eh?'

Here the storyteller peeks over the rim of his glasses and says theatrically: 'Yes. Dying from, ahem... a *respiratory* infection.'

Death cocooned in rumour and gossip...

But it was a time, like most times, like ours now, of great ignorance. I recall again seeing those first papers on AIDS in the *New England Journal of Medicine*. As said, I specifically remember thinking that the abstract had a misprint. That line about 1,000 partners a year. I thought maybe they meant ten, a hundred at a push. I – we – didn't have a clue: because of this ignorance, people died. Attitudes were slow to change.

Back in 1994 there was no HIV physician in Brighton. General and chest physicians looked after all these young people dying. Elton John would fund a centre for us in Brighton. Elton may well have gone out on a Saturday night in the '70s with a belly full of beer and a barrel full of monkeys to start some fights, but he had grown up now it was the '90s. By 1995 my colleague Martin Fisher was appointed. He would transform the care for HIV+ people in the city and gain great respect, national and international acclaim. Before he arrived too many people were dying. Young people we could do nothing for.

A small minority of doctors remain homophobic. Many of those double up as racist. There is a small group of reactionary, generally older physicians who will do their best to avoid seeing minority group patients at clinics, handing their care over to younger colleagues or registrars. And they are sly with it, never dropping their bourgeois guard enough to utter any epithet that might have them censured. As for trans patients: *You don't look after those, do you?*

One of the more distressing cases I dealt with was a trans woman, a healthcare worker. This was a gifted, caring person, who had heard, on many occasions, abuse from other members of staff. She reported this but came up against a brick wall of bureaucracy. The result, as is so often the case for whistle-blowers in the NHS, was unhelpful and traumatic.

We would appear to be living through times when these hatreds are coming back to the fore, legitimised by educated people who should know better. Educated people who seem to be living in the past, a past with servants and an empire: megalothymia.

Identity politics could cause issues when examining. The Royal College of Physicians exam is a global qualification: the MRCP. Part of the exam is called PACES (Practical Assessment of Clinical Examination Skills) and is held in various hospitals in the UK. The organisation of a PACES exam requires serious effort. One of the stations in the exam uses an actor to test communication skills. Those whose mother tongue is English are at a distinct advantage; those who have worked in the NHS even more so.

Two examiners, both senior consultants, both Fellows of the college, sit to one side and observe the interaction between the candidate and the actor playing a patient. Pass the exam and you are well on the way to becoming a consultant physician; fail the exam several times and you will not be one. The exam is costly, over £1,000 a go.

I've examined for twenty years now. With my co-examiner we meet with an actor, a young straight man who is to play a gay man who has come to get the result of an HIV test; he doesn't know it is positive. The first candidate comes into the room and performs well. She tells the actor the diagnosis with tact and sensitivity. The actor plays shock well. They go through the implications of the diagnosis and after the allotted twelve minutes the consultation is over, we ask her a few questions and then an assistant knocks our door at fourteen minutes. She can now leave to attend the other stations. We have a couple of minutes to mark and record any worries. The next candidate comes in.

He's a middle-aged man who might be from Saudi Arabia. He is courteous, caring, and he goes through the actor's history carefully. He clearly knows his task is to break the bad news. He's doing well and then this happens: 'I need to ask you some personal questions, is this all right?'

The actor nods, says: 'Sure.'

'You live here, yes?'

'Yes, I do. Is that relevant?'

'No, not really, I'm sorry. But maybe I can ask next: are you married?'

'Yes, I am.'

'And your wife. She well?'

'I don't have a wife.'

The candidate looks down at his notes, reads for a moment or two, looks up again: 'You are married, yes?'

'Yes.'

'Your wife, she is well, yes?'

'I don't have a wife.'

He looks down at his notes again, takes out a handkerchief, mops his brow, tries one more time: 'Your wife, you are married: your wife, she is keeping well?'

The actor is stony, impassive, in the role. He gives nothing away. Emphatically he now says: 'I've told you, I don't have a wife.'

The candidate looks up at the ceiling and now around the room, his gaze now settling on us, the two examiners, his eyes gently pleading for help, but we can give him none. We have to sit in painful silence for another eight minutes or so until that knock on the door. The instructions for the exam are very clear: we can say nothing. Eight long minutes. Eight minutes is a very long time when you desperately want to help someone who is clearly drowning. Eventually he leaves the room, broken.

At the wash-up session after with our fellow examiners from the other stations we discuss the passes and the failures. If someone has failed badly we decide if counselling is required. We discuss our case (he's failed badly on the other stations too) and a debate is had as to whether it is reasonable or unreasonable to fail someone on what can only be called cultural grounds. This poor lad was clearly unaware of British law on gay marriage: can he be faulted for that? Yes, we concluded, in a sense he can: we would expect cultural sensitivity to all patients regardless of race, creed or gender preference. He should have asked the actor for clarification, as simple as that, and he might have passed our station at least. We would certainly fail a UK-born candidate if they showed a Muslim patient a similar form of disrespect.

Examiners are scrutinised too: we are graded as hawks or doves, given the subsequent computerised interrogation of our marking data. Too predatory or too passive scoring can lead to remedial training or even removal as an examiner. Examiners can also behave badly. One elderly rake was upbraided a few years back by two of my female colleagues for inappropriate remarks about the fit of their clothing during an exam. And then there was the time our female registrar of the day helped us out.

Her parents were from Hong Kong. The lead examiner was taking us through the wash-up after the candidates had left. He was talking to the group of examiners about one of the candidates and described this woman as 'the one with the slanty eyes'. YOU WHAT?

I quickly saw the pained expression on my registrar's face after she heard this inanity. We had to pull the lead examiner out the room, tell him his error and insist he apologise to her *immediately* and confirm this in writing.

We're back on the wards down by the coast in the mid-1990s. I'm struck by how many of our patients with diabetes and foot ulcers are male. All seem to be men in their late fifties, early sixties, often living alone, often neglecting themselves. These are guys who do not have vascular disease (they have reasonable foot pulses), but they do have neuropathy, impaired sensation that has rendered their feet numb. They are vulnerable to injury from, say, a tack in their shoe, or a grandchild's stray piece of Lego. And then they end up in hospital for weeks on end treated with intravenous antibiotics, often bedbound for pressure relief to give the ulcer a chance to heal. They are guys like Mike.

Mike was nearing sixty, overweight, myopic and bald. He had a great booming laugh that would lighten his shining moon-face. Superficially he cut a jolly Falstaffian figure, but Mike was living in a world of pain. His dressings were taken down and I looked at the ulcer on the base of his foot. This looked pink and clean with no pus, no rank smell. Medicine remains (crucially) an olfactory discipline: if you are squeamish about smells then pick another career. I smiled up at Mike and said that I thought it looked better. He asked if I could speak with him after the ward round.

Later I head back alone: 'So, Michael, how can I help you?'

He looks at me intently with his eyes magnified by his thick lenses: 'I need to talk to you… confidentially.'

'Sure. This conversation will be private. What's up?'

'My foot. I'm going to lose it, right? Be straight with me.'

I express surprise: 'Your foot? No, no, I don't want you thinking that, Mike. You are not going to lose it.'

'Is that a promise?'

'Well… yes… I guess… yes, it is. That's a promise. Look, your circulation is excellent. We just need to keep the pressure off it for some time and it will heal. That's a promise.'

I see the relief on his face but something else as well, something darker perhaps. I look for a chink: 'There's something you're not telling me, isn't there, Mike? C'mon, out with it.'

He's hesitant. I haven't seen him so lacking in confidence before: 'I'm… I'm scared about my feet. Really scared.'

'Well, that's natural. None of us wants anything bad to happen to them. We need 'em both.'

'No. You don't understand. My feet… my feet have been hurt before.'

'What, hurt in an accident?'

'No… something else.'

His cagey replies are reflected in his furrowed brow, his gaze now downcast: 'Can I tell you something I've told only a few people?'

'Of course.'

'Well… you know I was a journalist. Am a journalist.'

'Yes, indeed. The team told me that you're the opera critic for the evening paper. That must be great. Do you get to Glyndebourne much?'

'I do, yes, I love it. But before that I was a war correspondent.'

I'm being very careful now. I pause and then say quietly, slowly: 'Right. I see. Can I ask where?'

'Vietnam. Angola.'

'Vietnam. The 'Nam! That must have been something, right?'

'Yeah, I had a wonderful time. Kind of. But it was Angola...' His voice tails off.

Then he tells me the full story. In Angola he was captured by the communist forces and assumed to be a British spy. He was tortured. His feet were beaten. And then he tells me that he has no time for doctors, no time at all, and that I will have my work cut out to gain his trust: 'Because it was doctors who tortured me. East German doctors.'

Slowly but surely over the next few weeks I try to impress upon him that we are on his side. We talk about opera: he knows his subject and has interviewed many divas. He urges me to go to Glyndebourne even though he knows I'm a philistine. We talk books. He loves Vasily Grossman's *Life and Fate*. He tells me that Stalin would have had me shot: 'You would have been one of the first. Doctors. Up against the wall.' Then came Mike's booming laugh.

I meet his estranged wife. She still cares for him but things have not been the same since Angola; in fact even further back, since Vietnam. She tells me he was injured in Vietnam but doesn't go into the details. He hasn't told me anything about that. After he is discharged, his ulcer healed, I see him at outpatients and he seems cheerier. He praises a soprano I haven't heard of and again pesters me to go and see some opera. He gives me some books he has reviewed, mainly thick historical tomes about the Cold War. I'm curious about his time in Vietnam: 'Did you know McCullin?'

'I did, yeah. And Page, Tim Page. He once asked a chopper crew to fly over a combat zone while he was suspended in some netting below the landing runners, spread-eagled, and then he was all snap, snap. He got some great shots. Mad as a hatter.'

'He was badly injured out there, wasn't he?'

'Yeah. And I was too. Stepped on a mine. End of my marriage.'

And then that deep laugh of his again.

He'd seen too much in Vietnam. He had stories about the VC using sharpened sticks, perforating eardrums. He knew of Errol Flynn's son, Sean, but didn't go motorcycling with him up to Hue. Didn't accompany Sean and Dana Stone into the deadly heart of darkness that was Khmer-era Cambodia. One day I asked him: 'How did you get into all this?'

He was quick to apportion blame: 'Hemingway. It was all Hem's fault. Papa. Crazy I know but I get angry at him sometimes because of what happened to me, the blast, the torture, all of it. As a young reporter I just loved Hem. I wanted to be like Papa. I wanted to get lost in the barrios, run with the bulls, catch fish and hunt big game. Generally I wanted to get into trouble in dangerous places. Grace under pressure and all that. Didn't quite work out that way.'

We became friends. I asked a colleague to look after him so that we could meet up for a drink, my professional duties now over. He liked asking my wife about midwifery. Childbirth cheered him. At base he remained an optimist despite his inner despair: *People will keep on having babies.* We would sometimes meet at the art deco aerodrome in Shoreham as light aircraft buzzed around us. He was hopeless with his diet; he loved zucchini fritters. His weight ballooned; his diabetes control worsened. Today he might have been offered bariatric surgery. His foot held: for that he was eternally grateful. But all the time I knew he was at a high risk of a heart attack or a stroke. And then one morning his wife called me. There would be no more exchanges of books on spies and spying, on Russia and the revolution.

His funeral was a humanist affair with time for people to head up to the pulpit and speak about him. I took my turn and stumbled out something about his love of Hemingway.

Medicine might appear to be a world of action. And it is for those working in dangerous parts of the planet faced with the likes of Ebola. Dangerous too, closer to home, in this age of Covid-19. I was more cowardly. I settled for the comforts of the south English coast. But Mike was a proper man of action. In a crazy way I'm envious of his mad life. Well, parts of it anyway. His stories still haunt me. I'm still very unsettled about East German doctors of a certain generation.

12

THE CLOT

Brighton. From the wards you can look directly out to sea: blue sea, blue sky. Yachts. The pier. I'm on our ward talking with a new colleague. He's ten years older than me, in his mid-forties. He was educated at a public school, Westminster, and went up to Oxford. Sometimes he says things like: 'Not everything about the empire was bad. Take the railway system in India, for example.'

He's a fine clinician and we spend time talking about our interesting cases over coffee. He's troubled this morning: 'What do you make of that new student?'

'What new student?'

'That elective lad, from up your way. Dundee, I think he said.'

Up my way. That's like saying Newcastle was down his way.

The elective period at medical school is during the third and fourth years when a student spends about six weeks working in a hospital for practical experience: they are usually encouraged to do these overseas, see the world a bit, get a more rounded picture of global health, suffering in the third world. But it takes money to go abroad and so hard-up students often end up doing these electives in UK hospitals. Excitable surgical wannabes go to America for gunshot experience. I did my electives in Reading and Colchester.

Who was this new student? I meet Pete on my next ward round. He introduces himself and confirms he is indeed at Dundee University. He's in his fourth year. His surname is odd: Fud.

'Fud?'

'Yes, but it's pronounced 'food'. Pete Fud.'

'Right.'

He's shitting me, surely? We press on. We meet the patients on the ward: a couple of new men with foot ulcers now that Mike has gone; three lonely elderly patients waiting for 'placement' – a nursing home, in other words; a young woman in early pregnancy who has diabetes and renal problems. I'm accompanied by one of the ward sisters, my house officer, a registrar and Fud. I turn to him: 'OK, Pete, tell me the six hormones made by the anterior pituitary.'

His smooth young face looks blank. Maybe he hasn't done any endocrinology yet. I give him a pass: 'Maybe you haven't done that in Dundee?'

He thinks he's off the hook.

'No, not yet.'

'OK, have a shot though. Think what the pituitary controls, what other organs it influences.'

I'm trying to help him. The educationalists have told us that the brow-beating style of instruction we were used to at medical school is old hat, insulting and, worse, ineffective as a learning strategy. Sometimes in the past we would be sent off ward rounds by our consultants and told to go to the library and not come back until we had mugged up on whatever it was we were supposed to master. There could be mocking laughter. A student in my year was with a professor on a round when they came to a patient with ketoacidosis.

The professor aimed a question at him. This in front of the large retinue of other students tagging along: 'So, what do you think this man's pH was when he arrived?'

The normal body pH is around 7.35–7.45. Life-threatening DKA may present with a pH just under seven. I have not seen anyone survive a pH under 6.7. The student answers confidently: '3.6.'

The professor is apoplectic: this is the pH of vinegar. 'WHAT! Did you say 3.6?'

'Yes, well, I didn't want to make him *too* acidotic.'

The poor guy was guffawed off the ward.

I try again with Fud: 'So, Pete, the pituitary makes hormones, right?'

'Yes.'

'And where do they act on? What other glands?'

'Glands?'

'Yes, Pete, what other glands?'

I'm beginning to lose patience, but he comes back with: 'The thyroid?'

'Yes! Correct, the thyroid. I knew you knew! Any others you might know?'

'The kidney?'

'The kidney? Well, the kidney can be seen as an endocrine organ but, no, the kidney is not really under *direct* anterior pituitary control. Look, Pete, read up on it before the next ward round, OK? And check out the posterior pituitary too. That's the bit that acts on the kidney. We need some coffee now to act on our kidneys, eh?'

I meet up with my older colleague again and we discuss Pete. He has reached a conclusion: 'He's rubbish, isn't he?'

My head answers yes, Fud is a dud. No one calls him 'food'. He's Fud as in crud. But maybe we should give Fud a chance. We agree.

We will reassess his performance at the end of the week. And then we titter again at his surname like a pair of schoolboys.

Next day I bump into a surgeon. He's narked about a long list of tiresome irritations (as surgeons often are), but suddenly his face brightens and, beaming now, says: 'That Fud student: is he one of yours? Fud! What a name! Isn't that what you people up north call…? Hope he doesn't want to become a gynaecologist. Jeez, he's hopeless. Knew nothing about anatomy. And I mean nothing!'

I walk down one of the long windowless white corridors in the hospital, my heels click-clicking again like Lee Marvin from *Point Blank*. Just like Lee: like a pissed-off Lee. And I'm thinking hard. Thinking about Pete and that kidney comment. I meet again with my senior colleague and start our reassessment: 'He *really* knows nothing.'

'I know.'

'I just met one of the surgeons and he thought it was funny. But it isn't. Not really.'

'No.'

'I mean, Dundee. Wonder why he decided to study up there?'

'Are you thinking what I'm thinking?'

We stare at one another, contemplating the worst. I make a suggestion: 'Maybe we should phone medical staffing.'

I give them a call and they check on Pete Fud. Yes, they tell me, he's from Dundee University: 'We have a letter from them confirming he is one of their students.'

So that's all right then. But later, over yet another coffee, our team is talking about him again. Fud knows f-all. We've talked to the registrar, our houseman and the ward sister. And they're all worried about him too. I decide to call Dundee direct.

They've never heard of him.

They tell me to wait a second.

They sent a letter of rejection to him three years ago.

I quickly call medical staffing and tell them this: they look again at his letter. It's a cut-and-paste job. He's a fraud. He is not a medical student. And he's running around our hospital right now examining people. There's only one way forward. We call the police.

Pete was cautioned. His real name wasn't Fud. We learned later that his mum and dad were professionals of some sort. The poor kid was under intense paternal pressure to succeed.

I was now in my forties: I didn't watch medical shows on TV any more. Since I stopped watching endless reruns of *M*A*S*H* I've avoided American shows like *ER* (I don't like A+E much in real life so why should I want to spend my free time in a virtual equivalent?) or their UK siblings: *Casualty*, *Holby City* and *Cardiac Arrest*. My colleagues tell me how life-like *Cardiac Arrest* is. Joshing stories about catheter bags filled with cold tea. *You should really watch it, you'd love it.* But I've heard that the writer has now left medicine, disillusioned, gone before even trying to become a senior clinician. I don't want that to happen to me. I'm keen to keep some of my illusions, at least for now. My old headmaster used to say: *There's nothing sadder than a teenage cynic.* Let's extend that – maybe there's nothing sadder than the under-fifty-year-old doctor as cynic. How long did the writer, Jed Mercurio, stick it out? The fans of the show tell me Jed left medicine *before* becoming a registrar. I'm irrationally annoyed again but in truth deeply jealous of Jed Mercurio. I'd love to take some time off and write. It would be great to get some of the stories I've heard down on paper.

What patients said when you were taking blood in the days before hospitals employed venesectors. A lady from Fulking: 'Oops-a-dai-sy: here comes the vampire!'

A man exiled from Manchester: 'Is me blood going off t' black pudding factory then?'

A pensioner originally from Belfast: 'You must 'ave buckets of it buh neu.'

Some of the older patients would remember that unfunny Tony Hancock line about wanting an armful. They'd say: 'Just like Tony Hancock.' I cannot imagine this line ever being funny. An armful. *And?* What, exactly, is funny about that? I'm really missing something here, but then I'm not a fuckin' comedian. Hancock was. Then he killed himself. I watched old YouTube footage of him being interviewed on *Face to Face.* He was a sad mess of a man. Watching the clip is intensely painful, like being a voyeur at a psychiatric con-sultation. Comedians can be fucking depressing.

I lost count of how many times I had the following exchange: 'Right, shoes and socks off, let me examine your feet.'

The man is from Edinburgh, his voice like a pedantic newscaster: 'What, both of them?'

I'm still trying to understand what patients really meant by saying that. Did they think that one foot was as good as another? Maybe they thought they were trying to be funny like Tony Hancock. Trying to get a laugh. Patients who fancy themselves as comedians: this is one of the great medical challenges doctors face daily. You make a noise at their punchline, which sounds something like *nneugh.* A non-laugh thing that might be taken for assent but really means this: shut up please. These fuckin' comedians are the sorts who call you by your first name, like a guy from Peacehaven who comes to see me: *Hatch right, John. How are you today, John? Do whatever you say, John. 'Ello, John, got a new motor!'* Heh, heh, heh, heh, huh.

My interior monologue insistently, loudly, now rants: WHEN DID I SAY YOU COULD CALL ME JOHN?

It's Doctor Quin to you, mate. But I don't utter this out loud because if I had he'd say this: 'Ah, rightchar! Just like Dr Quinn, medicine woman! Are you any relative then?'

At first monthly, then weekly, then daily, the comedians would ask me: 'Oh! So… are you related to Dr Quinn, medicine woman?'

Reader, I married her. I'd spin this yarn: 'Yeah, we got divorced. Jane. She's a lovely woman. Sad that we broke up. Did you see her in *Live and Let Die*? Solitaire…'

After about five years of this on a nearly daily basis (I'm now the wrong side of forty-five) the darkly impatient part of my brain is saying: *Tell them to fuck the fuck off.*

I don't say it. You don't say that out loud. But Danvers does. Danvers phones me out of the blue from Glasgow one night. A junkie on a ward round had been pestering him for some methadone. Whining away at him. So Danvers told him to fuck right off. Right there on the ward. And… nothing happened. The junkie shut up. Maybe that's the difference between being a doctor in Glasgow and being one in the south of England. In Glasgow you can tell someone acting up to fuck off. Down here you can't. Down here your arse wouldn't touch the ground. Down here it would be P45 time.

My colleague is telling me about the patients on the wards, the ones that I am about to inherit from him. This is the handover. One of them is a woman in her early fifties who has presented with a seizure. My colleague thinks that she has had a stroke. Thrombolytic (clot-busting) drugs are a long way off in the future and I'm told that the prognosis for the poor woman is bleak. We are still in the twentieth century. Intensive care are now involved in her management:

they are in charge. I go and see her there because if she recovers she will come back to my ward and my care; this is how it works. She lies quietly on the bed, pitifully weak down her left-hand side. She has had a CT scan and the neuroradiologists have reported the images as being consistent with a stroke. The ITU team has spoken with her family; they have not been optimistic. I suggest we get the neurologists to see her and they duly arrive and concur with the diagnosis. They order an MRI scan of the brain and again the consultant neuroradiologists say the appearances are consistent with a stroke.

Some days pass and her condition deteriorates. She has further visits from the neurologists and has two more scans, all of which are reported to be consistent with a diagnosis of stroke. And then she dies.

A month later and, out of the blue while I'm doing a clinic, a pathologist phones and asks if I knew this woman and her case. I tell him I did and he says swiftly: 'She had an abscess. A brain abscess. That's what killed her.'

A minority of pathologists are not that concerned about the impact their news might have on the clinician: if we have got it wrong then, well, that's for us, the clinicians, to deal with.

I feel sick to the pit of my stomach. I count in my head. She saw at least six consultants, two of whom are consultant neurologists, God knows how many 'junior' doctors, had four scans reviewed by another two consultant neuroradiologists... and we still got it wrong. We all got it wrong. If it had been diagnosed she could have had surgery, she might have lived...

I call up the senior neurologist. We agree on what we have to do. We have to meet up with the family. We have to tell them the truth.

We sit with them in a quiet room. Her parents are still in deep bereavement. They know we want to discuss the post-mortem re-sults. Our words come out carefully, steadily, but when I speak I feel as if my throat is tightening. Telling the truth can be very hard when it implicates you and all your team in failure. And when we tell them what was found they are... silent. They understand what we are saying to them. We got it wrong. The silence is long. The unsaid is being thought by them and by us. Will we be able to carry on as doctors? Will we lose our jobs, our vocation? Inside I'm shak-ing. We explain our rationale for thinking that she had had a stroke. We go through the scans. We apologise once, twice, three, many many times. We cannot apologise enough. We express our disap-pointment that sometimes we are only as good as our technology if the scans point us in the wrong direction.

Mistakes are made every day in medicine. We try to reduce these as much as we can, systems can always improve, but we will never be right 100 per cent of the time. Medicine will always pose serious challenges. If we were to fire every doctor who made a mistake, we would have no doctors. Never-events, that's what they call them now – events that should never happen. But with cutbacks in the service it is hard to see how we can prevent these from happening.

I find myself apologising for the service every day. Sometimes I'm apologising hourly. My dreams are full of apologies. *I'm sorry*. I'm really sorry.

A Sunday afternoon, a day off, and I sit reading at home. The phone rings and it is Raymond. Raymond is a senior cardiologist, one of the cool, and one of the most capable doctors in the hospital. He projects calm, common sense. He rarely phones me and when he does it is for a very good reason. The last time he called it was about his dog. This poor creature was going hypoglycaemic and it turned out to have a pancreatic tumour producing excess insulin, an insulinoma. These are extremely rare: in humans maybe one in a million. I've looked after no more than five people in my career with the great misfortune to have an insulinoma. Most are benign, but sometimes radical surgery, the dreaded Whipple's procedure, is required. The word 'Whipple's' strikes fear into most doctors. A Whipple's is a brutal operation that entails much chopping and binning of organs. Complications are common. I dread to think what Raymond ended up paying his vet. Anyway, this Sunday the conversation was very different: 'Afternoon, JDQ, greetings from Worthing.'

'Hi Raymond, what takes you over to that world of wonders?'

'Well, I have a lady on the angio table here who came in a couple of hours ago with some chest pain... but her coronaries are clean. There is, though, a large blush in her abdomen and I think this might be right up your *strasse*.'

This is how a clever cardiologist tells an endocrinologist that what we are dealing with here is another of those rare tumours that somehow contrive to present on a weekend when consultants are supposed to be out golfing. Raymond thinks that lady has a phaeo. Fee-oh. A phaeochromocytoma: wonderful word. Phaeos are tumours of the adrenal glands that, like insulinomas, are often 'benign'. That's benign as in rarely metastatic; however, these tumours are anything but benign in their effects. By secreting large volumes of adrenaline, spikes of high-octane hormone, angina can be induced (coronary ischaemia) and that can be quite fatal.

Phaeos scare doctors and rightly so: they scare the hell out of me. Anaesthetists sometimes discover one with serendipity when actively intra-operative. Serendipity: discovered by chance in a happy or beneficial way. Beneficial for the patient, sure, once removed. But you wouldn't describe the anaesthetist as 'happy' at this precise moment. They find to their horror that a patient's blood pressure becomes spectacularly labile – up and down like the Big Dipper at the end of Brighton Pier. The anaesthetist puts away the pink *FT* they've been scanning. This is one of the rare times an endocrinologist gets called to an operating theatre.

We transfer the lady across from Worthing. On arrival I see a middle-aged woman who looks very pale; she is invaded in multiple places by plastic lines. She's in trouble. Her heart rate is racing and I'm thinking we need to slow it *right* down but then she does this by herself and goes too far; she arrests. She is asystolic. Some might call that 'dead'. Her blood pressure is now nil; seconds earlier it was as high as the Himalayas. We get her rhythm back after a thump, and with the help of the anaesthetist we start her on a drug I have only rarely had to call on: sodium nitroprusside. Like insulin, this drug has a very short intravenous half-life and so we can switch off its effect quickly. The woman looks ghastly and I'm reminded that nitroprusside as a substance is allied to cyanide. She arrests again and there's more thumping on her chest and more cardioversion, more shocks from the defibrillator. That life of action, Mike's kind of life, Mike and his derring-do in the 'Nam: here was another variant.

The woman stabilises and the next day we get her to the scanner: this confirms she has a huge tumour above her left kidney. Ten centimetres in size: this just *has* to be a phaeo. We then dampen down the effect of the excess adrenaline, and we do this with a drug called phenoxybenzamine. This is another drug we very rarely use and as a result there is not infrequently a supply problem. Thankfully we have some today and we load her. It takes a couple of weeks to fully prepare the lady for surgery, but she gets through it safely and afterwards I pop down to theatre to meet the surgeon, who plonks the tumour proudly into my gloved hands, like a cat who has captured a magpie and brought it home to its disbelieving owner. It's out. She will live.

I follow her up annually and each year for fifteen years she gives me a big hug as she leaves. Medicine can be fantastic. A friend bested this story and told me recently about another phaeochromocytoma case; this time the tumour was embedded in the heart. The surgeons took the heart out, as if in preparation for a transplant, and got the patient on extracorporeal circulation. They then carefully dissected the tumour out of the isolated heart on a table away from the patient and carefully put the now tumour-free organ back in place. Sci-fi stuff.

It's the first morning of the junior doctors' strike. The GMC are now saying that some junior doctors could get struck off if they down tools for five days. Their war with the government continues.

New to Brighton, I'm invited to join what I suspect to be a secret society after another unexpected phone call. I'm told the society has no name. A distinguished voice at the end of the line says: 'It's called the Innominate Society. After the bone, the hip, you understand? They couldn't think of a name when it was started, hence innominate...'

Turns out it's not a secret society. I learn that the Innominate has been going since 1860 or thereabouts, so maybe it might be hip to join, hip to join the Innominate. Bad gag. There are sixteen members: eight GPs and eight hospital consultants. I think fourteen men and only two women at that time. Once retired, you drop out. New members are selected on one criterion: 'Can you tell us a good story?'

The meetings are held monthly and rotate around each person's house. You meet and greet from 8 p.m., eat at 9 p.m. (so potentially you need to cater for sixteen people) and then you talk from ten to ten-thirty. The group then discusses the matter in hand for another half an hour; we head home at eleven. The voice on the line goes on: 'Wine will be drunk. You can talk about anything you like but most pick a topic that is vaguely to do with medicine. Colin did one on bees recently.'

To refuse would appear churlish in the face of such generosity. And as someone new to the area I crave some sense of inclusion. I sign up. My wife, like most of the partners of the members, is less than pleased about the catering issue. In time this will be addressed. In time too the dress code changes from suit and tie to jeans and T-shirts. The ratio of male to female corrects itself to 1:1. The food is demoted from attempts to plate up a three-course feast to dishing out more basic fare. The wine remains a constant.

Dylan is one of the older members and he's a child psychiatrist; he looks after the boys at Eton. He tells us that the headmaster has invited us over for dinner in order that we visit the library and see some of William Harvey's original drawings of the circulation. There is some debate amongst the younger members, the liberals from Lewes and the more urban leftists, of the group. We decide to go. My own conclusion is that I should see with my own eyes what I have been brought up by Orwell to distrust: make up my own mind.

We arrive in a hired coach and duly visit the library. The Harveian drawings are exquisitely detailed and impressive: well worth the trip. There are photographs too of various explorers and heroes like T. E. Lawrence and Wilfred Thesiger. Pictures taken with the 'natives': a deluded vision of supremacy that would crash down on Britain in the future. Megalothymia.

The headmaster is charming, a good dinner companion. He's an enthusiast in conversation, an explainer, but then what would you expect? He's a *teacher*. Later I get talking to his wife, who constantly fiddles with her hair. She tells me scattered factoids about the works of art that line the walls of the dining room. She asks if I noted the caricatures that line the corridor. I have. Old boys; many have been PM. Men who once ruled a quarter of the planet. Hard not to reflect on how debased the role has become these days. She asks if I know anything about the contemporary art market, because Jay Jopling from the blue-chip White Cube gallery has been with some of the older boys today. Sixteen-year-olds getting tips on what art to buy, whom to collect.

On leaving, we shake hands and thank the pair for a pleasant meal. I have no memory of what we ate or drank so I must assume it was relatively modest. I'm almost convinced of the goodness of Eton by their performance, but then this happens. As we cross the darkened quadrangle on our way back to the coach, I notice some objects on the grass, scattered flat things: what could they be? I bend and pick one up: it's a jotter. The quadrangle is littered with pupils' jotters. Why?

An elderly man in a uniform passes and I ask him cheerily: 'What's this all about then?'

'What? Oh, those! That's the senior boys, they leave them for the fags, the juniors, to pick up.'

'Right. The fags.'

On the trip back the Innominate group oohs and aahs about the Harvey manuscripts; a minority tacitly blesses the school and all that it stands for. I say nothing about those jotters.

A month later and I'm in A+E again and the registrar rushes up to me. He's got a young woman in resus and isn't sure what to do next: 'She's in some sort of SVT but hasn't responded to adenosine.'

Her heart rate is racing and the standard cardiological remedy for a supraventricular tachycardia hasn't worked. We have a better drug now than verapamil, the one I used back in my Glasgow days, back when we did fast atrial pacing, back with Harty, the pipe-smoking cardiologist. The registrar shows me the ECG and I'm thinking, yes, that's fast, maybe we should get our non-pipe-smoking cardiologists down.

'How old is she?'

'Nineteen.'

'Let's go and see her.'

She looks like shit and I'm immediately scared. She's pale, clammy and looks very, very frightened. She knows she is dying and I do too. This is not an SVT. Her systolic blood pressure is low, around seventy. She is shocked and she is blue and she is very breathless. Nurses and doctors surround her and we need an answer. We need an answer now.

I examine her very quickly: she has breath sounds in both lung fields so she does not have an obvious pneumothorax, and it's not a haemopneumothorax either, like that young girl years ago back in Glasgow. Memories of the past are crucial in medicine. Have I seen this before? What did we do then? Her abdomen is soft and non-tender and so there appears to be no gross surgical problem. I'm told swiftly that she is not pregnant because she is on the pill, a test is pending, and that there is no history of bleeding.

I'm looking at her legs and one looks a little swollen. I ask her to nod or shake her head when I ask: 'Is your leg sore?'

I look up and see that the faces of the other carers are now lit up like neon strip-lights with recognition. She's got a clot in her leg and it has gone to her lung. She's got a PE, a pulmonary embolism, probably related to being on the pill, a rare but well-known complication. We need to confirm the diagnosis by putting her through the CT scanner and getting some dye into her pulmonary arteries to identify if there is a clot there.

But there's one other diagnosis that can cause a similar kind of picture, much rarer than a PE, and that is a dissection of the aorta. I've seen this happen a couple of times: once in an older man with high blood pressure, the other time in a tall thin man, a basketball player, who had Marfan syndrome. Marfan's is a condition that can weaken the lining of the aorta, the main blood vessel from the heart, the body's main highway, its M1. The girl is not tall, not thin. The CT will differentiate between them both. You've got to discriminate between these diagnostic possibilities because the clot-buster treatment for a PE will kill someone with a dissection: 'Let's get her to the scanner.'

'We don't have time.'

The head nurse is adamant and he's right. The girl is about to arrest. We have to treat her *now*. He draws up one of the newer clot-busting drugs. He hands the loaded syringe to the registrar: 'Shall I give it?'

He's asking me. If it is a PE it should save her. If it is an aneurysm the anticoagulation effect will kill her. Such a choice has never been as stark in my career. I have to make my mind up. Right. This. Second.

We give it.

And we watch. Seconds, minutes, pass.

And then the collective relief in seeing her blood pressure come up. She doesn't arrest. Fifteen minutes in and her breathing is now easing too. And I can feel the clamminess in my armpits: 'Let's get her to the scanner.'

The CT confirms it is a PE: there is a whopper of a clot blocking the blood from her heart getting to the lungs, where it is oxygenated. I think: *She's going to make it.* The team wheels her back into resus and we call ITU, who agree to take her when they can get a bed. Getting beds is getting harder and harder these days. Numbers are down: this stresses us out. All of us: the carers, the managers. And nationally it is getting worse. Beds are scarce. People talk of 'at-risk' discharges.

About ten minutes after the girl returns to resus I'm called urgently to see her again. Fuck. She's gone back to the way she was when I
first saw her about an hour ago. She's dying: she's dying again.

I'm trying to think fast while I watch her go a deeper shade of blue
despite the oxygen, despite the clot-busting drug. She's near purple.
Could she have an aneurysm after all? No, the radiologist was certain. And I've seen the filling defect myself on the scan confirming
she has a clot. OK, try to calm down: what should we do now?

Can we give her more of the clot-busting drug? There's a pharmacist at hand. I ask them, hoping against hope they will say yes,
yes, try it again. But they shake their head. No. You've given her the
correct dose. There's no evidence giving any more will work.

OK: second thought. The surgeons!

I call the cardiothoracic registrar, stressing the urgency of the
situation: can he cut it out?

'You've given her thrombolysis, right? If I cut her she'll bleed to
death.'

And with that he hangs up.

Third thought? Give me a third solution: please, God, please.

As I stand watching her sink, a thought arrives from somewhere.
A memory of something I've read in a textbook, a journal? A
memory of another case I've heard about? I call Phil, the cardiologist on call. Can he come in and see her and maybe manipulate a
catheter into her heart and, well, can he try to suck the clot out, or
break it up, or something, anything?

I'm desperate with worry. She's nineteen. I can see her eyes now,
she's pleading at me, give me more life.

Phil comes in quickly, gets her prepped and inserts a line. He
removes fifteen centimetres of clot. And she lives. Phil has saved
her.

13

FORMULA ONE AND CHEKHOV

Liam Farrell is a retired GP who used to work in the Armagh border town of Crossmaglen and is a long-standing contributor to the *British Medical Journal*. He writes wisely and well. He *is* a fuckin' comedian. I follow him on Twitter and see this morning he mentions a paper in the *British Journal of Urology*. The report suggests that men who ejaculate more than five times a week reduce their risk of prostatic cancer by a third. I tell my wife this and tweet her response (privately) to Liam. She says: 'I guess I'll have to take that on the chin.'

In my late thirties, inspired by Liam's writings, I send a pitch to *The Lancet*. They take it and I complete my first review of an art show: James Gillray caricatures then on display at St Bart's. *The Lancet* publish the piece in 2000 with the dreadfully punning title 'Look back at Ingres'. Soon after, I get another stroke of luck and publish another review, this time of a biography of Vera Nabokov in *The Guardian*. I get the bug.

I'm reading a short story by the young Chekhov called 'Chase Two Rabbits, Catch None' that appeared in 1880. I think he was twenty at the time and a medical student. Maria Bloshteyn writes that 'he apparently saw personal meaning in the proverb as he saw himself as chasing after two rabbits, as it were, of medicine and writing'. Chekhov himself wrote: 'That proverb about the two rabbits drove me to the point of insomnia.' It gets me thinking too.

I've been seeing Stuart for a decade. He first came to see me when he was in his mid-seventies because he'd been feeling tired; his libido was low. Could it be something to do with hormones? His morning testosterone was down, but then that's often the case in mid-seventies men; indeed, some of my peers wouldn't even have measured it. Most would have checked out other causes for tiredness but if any mention of testosterone treatment arose some would council great caution and send him on his way.

Studies on hormone replacement in elderly men are still somewhat in their infancy. The so-called 'andropause' remains a controversial concept. Many think that we should not interfere with the slow age-related decline in testosterone; there's a worry about the risk of prostatic cancer. Testosterone doesn't appear to *cause* prostatic cancer, but if you are unlucky enough to get prostate cancer then exogenous testosterone can worsen the situation. Prostatic cancer cells are stimulated by testosterone. Indeed, testosterone antagonists are one of the mainstays of prostate cancer therapy.

Stuart has read all this and he doesn't mind: he wants to be on testosterone replacement. He is prepared to take the risk. He wants to try the gel preparation. He knows that oral versions are hopeless. And he's not so keen on the three-monthly injections but he's willing to try this if all else fails.

Stuart is clearly highly educated. I ask what he used to do: 'You're assuming I've retired.'

'You're still working?'

'Oh yes.'

'Doing what, can I ask?'

'I'm supervising two PhD students.'

Turns out he is an Italianist. We agree to a trial of testosterone and I document that I've explained the risks. We meet every three months to assess his progress and monitor his blood PSA (prostate-specific antigen, a marker for prostate cancer) and haemoglobin. Excess testosterone can cause polycythaemia: thick blood. The treatment works and he's much happier. I get to know him. With each visit he impresses me more and more as a *mensch*.

He is from the north, Angus to be precise, and his accent is soft and gently authoritative. I've met not a few people from the Highlands who have moved south to great success. They epitomise J. M. Barrie's comment: 'There are few more impressive sights in the world than a Scotsman on the make.' Square that when it comes to the bright progeny of the Highlands and Islands. No, cube it.

Stuart tells me he has translated Pasolini's Friulian poems, Dino Buzzati's brilliant novel *The Tartar Steppe*, and Aldo Busi's racy *The Standard Life of a Temporary Pantyhose Salesman*. I tell him of my love for Moravia and Calvino, Bertolucci's *Novecento* and *Il conformista*. I study him carefully. He sits very still and looks at me with deep concentration. There's something of the Viking elder about him: full head of white hair, thick white eyebrows, a pronounced, intimidatory brow. He reminds me of my bridge inspector father-in-law. Stuart chooses his words carefully: unlike me he is no chatterer. I ask him about Edinburgh in the 1950s when he was mingling with the greats of Scottish literature: 'MacDiarmid? He could talk the hind legs off a donkey!'

'So why the Italian interest?'

'I was a POW during the war, but I escaped. Headed north. Joined the partisans.'

I try hard to curb my enthusiasm, but I want to hear more: jeez, this guy sitting in front of me is Von Ryan himself, he's been Frank Sinatra in a leather flying jacket, the Sinatra who hijacked a train heading north to Switzerland and freedom in *Von Ryan's Express*. Later, much later, I learn that Stuart was indeed in Army Intelligence.

Stuart knows his Marx, his Gramsci. The greats of Italian literature, their thoughts, their quotes trip off his tongue. He does this in a manner not meant to impress: this is the clear water of thought he swims in. He tells me about his impressive career with the BBC after the war. Controller of TV (no less) in 1963: he's the man who gave Britain *TWTWTW, That Was the Week That Was*.

And he wrote. He gives me a copy of his book *Carlino*. My wife and I read it a month or so later when we're on holiday in Liguria. *Carlino* is a barely concealed autobiographical account of Stuart's years with the partisans. In one tense and horrible scene a traitor is identified and the British man who has joined the group is tasked with shooting him.

When I return from our beautiful walks around Camogli and Portofino and I see him again at the clinic I'm emboldened to ask: 'That was you, wasn't it?'

He nods.

This man, this patient of mine, has just admitted to carrying out an execution. His silence is long. I've uncovered a seam of deep sadness. He has been haunted by these events for many years. After what seems an age, he goes on to tell me a story that suggests that there is persistent nobility in our world. Four decades later, hearing of his guilt and suffering, the mayor of the Italian town near where the incident took place got in touch with him. The town wanted

Stuart to visit and meet the family of the man he killed. The family wanted to forgive him publicly. He went over. The family told him that what he had done was terrible but correct. The man he shot was indeed a spy, was indeed a Fascist. The traitor would have had the group wiped out. And it was wartime.

Stuart tells me all this in the small clinic room with its rusty filing cabinets, its examination couch, its posters detailing different types of insulin. He speaks slowly with no drama, no romance. This is a secular confession. He is an agnostic. Stuart agrees with Nietzsche that God is dead.

Years later I read his obituary in *The Guardian*. Talking of his time with the partisans, he is quoted as saying: 'If I go back to Tuscany, I ask myself, "Well, was it worth it? To establish all these holiday homes?"... On the other hand, fascism lost.'

On his last ever visit to see me he was clearly quite frail, and before he died I asked him who he was currently reading: 'Back to the classics, my favourite: Horace.'

Stuart was probably the most impressive person I've ever met. This is what medicine, Chekhov's other rabbit, can offer you as a doctor: a sense that, as a profession, we have access to the inner worlds of others, other lives, other ways of being. And we will meet people who can say, with utter conviction because they enabled it to happen with dire acts, that fascism lost.

I call in the next patient and introduce myself. The lady is over-weight and waddles slowly to the chair. She beams when she hears my name: 'Oh! Just like Dr Quinn, medicine woman!'

Another medical conference. Medical conferences can be a dis-piriting experience. A near-constant drip-feed of corporate cyn-icism seemingly designed to lower the spirits. You find yourself confronting a naff 360-degree surround-sound screen advertising a drug with minimal advantage over a rival. You are jostled, bumped and pushed by colleagues from all over the planet, each desperate to collect the trashy freebies being handed out. As the years pass, I reduce the numbers of conferences I go to, ditch listening to Chuck thanking his family on Nantucket Island, his dog Jeb, *named after my favourite governor.* I prefer attending our specialty's European annual meeting when I can get to it. One in particular was special: Prague 1991, post-Velvet Revolution.

The combined effects of my fear of flying and the chance to travel overland behind the recently fallen Wall gave Cycling Scott and I the excuse to go by train. I recall spending an age at the border checkpoint in Cheb staring at the weeds between the railway tracks. I had a Sony Walkman playing The Orb's druggy instrumental 'O. O. B. E.'. Blankly looking out at the sidings, the grey huts devoid of humanity, the music seemed particularly appropriate, as with its title: Out-of-Body Experience. Hours later we chugged into the city. Free Prague itself retained its mystical aura, a medieval gloom that, particularly of an ill-lit night, recalled spooky Jewish tales featuring the Golem. Back then there were very few adverts plastering the walls; no Segways darting over the Charles Bridge; no daffy zorbs bouncing on the Vltava, no river of tourists in the Staré Město.

Walking around as the sun set, as your shadow lengthened, it was easy to conjure up the ghost of Kafka fretting about his father, imagining life as an insect. But there was an optimism in the moist air above the winding river below the unapproachable castle. Havel was President. A neon red love heart (designed by the artist Jiří David) would, in time, be installed over the government buildings: a cheeky reference to both redundant communist iconography and the, now-rampant, sex industry. David was implying the city had become an enormous brothel.

But in 1991 drunken British stag parties were not, as yet, omnipresent. We diabetologists were in the avant-garde of the Western invasion. We were about to discover that a pint of Budvar, a pint of Pilsner Urquell, cost eight pence.

We dined together, a gang of about twenty of us, gorging on pig shoulder and dumplings. Kris cut into one of his dumplings and found... raspberry jam. The total bill was under £20: a quid a head. We knew we should try to control ourselves, we knew we were ambassadors for our country, we were professionals... we should exercise constraint. But constraint goes out the window when beer is 8p a pint. By ten that evening the entire British contingent was unsteady. Discussions about new forms of insulin were slurred. No one was talking about IGFBP-5. We found a jazz club. And then a dark green bottle with a yellow label appeared: Becherovka.

'This cost 15p. Thought I would try it.'

This was Steve from Cambridge, the professor of medicine. The bottle was passed round the club. Scott, Kris, Martin: we all sipped tentatively and tasted... oil of cloves. This immediately conjured up memories of severe toothache, plugs of cotton wool dipped in oil of cloves. Scottish dentistry. Scottish dentistry after a childhood eating Oddfellows: pill-shaped confectionery tasting of... oil of cloves.

I looked at the locals in the club as a saxophone wailed. Czech men looked like the Beatles – the Beatles circa 1964, that is, with mop-top haircuts and cheap grey suits. And Czech girls wore purple miniskirts not seen on British streets since 1969. They reminded me of Bernadette Devlin. I thought of Milan Kundera and his cast of Czech surgeons, medics kicked out of their jobs by the communist regime only to end up cleaning windows: Kundera's naughty tales of fucking-as-displacement-activity. Prague's joyless anomie since the Soviets invaded: but what of now, what did 'freedom' offer? Drunken British diabetologists.

Richard has been seeing me regularly for years now at the clinic. He has autoimmune problems; his body is making antibodies against itself. He does not worry about the existential implications of this diagnosis (*I'm destroying myself? Ah well*). As a successful local businessman, he is more concerned about remembering to give himself insulin for his diabetes. Usually he does remember. He also has an underactive thyroid gland (he takes thyroxine) and Addison's disease, for which he takes replacement steroid.

He knows the sick-day rules for steroids: he knows to double his dose when he is unwell; he knows to attend A+E if he is vomiting and can't keep his steroids down. He proudly waves the copy of a letter I've sent him, with instructions for A+E if he is admitted, that he has now proudly laminated. Richard dresses neatly: suit and tie, polished shoes; he has the whole 'You can trust me with your money' businessman look. His manner is similarly sober, his face open, his hair cut neatly. He has a sly wit. He has a wife; he has children. I enjoy our chats. And then one morning I get a call to see him in ITU.

Why is he in intensive care? They tell me he was not in keto-acidosis; he was not in Addisonian crisis. The story was that his marriage was in trouble. Richard then drove off the cliffs high above the marina. I stare incredulously at the nurse who tells me this: 'And he survived!'

'As you can see...'

The cliff drop is at least a hundred feet. He's broken several bones and has sustained a severe head injury. I picture the car crashing through the barrier high above the sea, the sickening tilt of the vehicle at the edge, and then the fast fall to the under-hill walk. I see the car in my mind as it drops past the white chalk walls of the cliffs. I can picture the smash as it hits the ground, the sound of breaking glass, the impact of metal on concrete. And I look at Richard lying there; tubes coming out of his nose, his mouth; his fixed respirations, his chest moving steadily as controlled by the ventilator. He's pink, so his circulation must be fine. My eyes scan up to the monitors and see that his blood pressure and pulse are good too. His bloods are also reasonable: the team on ITU has his diabetes under control with an infusion of insulin; they've given him extra hydrocortisone intravenously to cover his Addison's. Amazingly he's going to pull through. I ask the nurse: 'But his head injury?'

'Bad.'

She shows me his CT brain scan images. They look awful. I'm not called back to see him again. There's talk of neuro-rehabilitation. Months and months and months pass and then one afternoon I'm called another time to A+E: 'There's a man here who says he knows you. Says you'd want to see him. He's waving a laminated letter around and it has your signature on it.'

It's Richard: he's survived! He's run out of insulin and it's a simple job to go and prescribe him some. I head down to see him, and my first impression is that he's looking great. His face beams with recognition as I arrive: 'I forgot to get more insulin, Dr Quin.'

'That's all right, Richard, we can sort that out. I'm amazed that you're OK! How long have you been out of hospital? Have you noticed any problem with your memory since the accident?'

'Yeah, I have, in fact. It's nowhere near as good.'

'Are you back at work yet?'

'No, they've given me some time off.'

He tells me he is now divorced. He has limited access to the children and is not allowed to take them out unaccompanied since the accident. As we talk, it becomes clearer that his memory, his short-term memory, has been seriously damaged: 'Where are you living now, Richard?'

'I can't remember the address, it's on this bit of paper.'

He's in digs and shows me a crumpled piece of scrap on which he has scrawled a street name. His writing seems to have deteriorated too. We agree on a time to meet again at my clinic. He duly forgets to attend.

Eventually he turns up a few months later at A+E to pick up another prescription for insulin and agrees, yet again, to come back to see me at outpatients and then, yet again, he forgets. This pattern continues for about another six months. The A+E staff tell me that he attends frequently, at other times out of standard working hours, waving my letter and demanding extra steroid; he swears at them if there is any delay. He wasn't like that before the accident. His personality has been damaged too. I somehow manage to get a hold of him and convince him to see me later that day at the clinic.

He sits in front of me in the room and it is immediately apparent that he has deteriorated in a very bad way since the crash. His hair is all over the place and unwashed. He is unshaven and looks spaced out as if high on dope. His sandshoes are stained and untied. His T-shirt has old bits of food stuck here and there. His memory is shot. He can remember my name but none of his recent hospital attendances.

'Where are you living now, Richard?'

'In the country.'

'That's nice. What, in a flat?'

'No. In a tent.'

'A tent!'

I'm appalled. We are in the early twenty-first century with the internet and billionaires, and this man who used to be a successful person is now, in his early forties, reduced to living in a tent near the cliffs where he had tried to commit suicide not more than a year before. I contact the social services. They say they will get on to it. But over the next six months I see Richard again and again and it becomes apparent that the social care network is failing him. Another year passes. He's still in the tent and he is refusing to be rehoused.

The winter arrives and the temperature drops and it snows. I go on holiday. When I return I learn that Richard was found dead in his tent. The pathologists think that he'd been dead for some time. This is Britain in the twenty-first century with its Wi-Fi, its Twitter, Facebook, Apple products, easyJet holidays, Amazon and Starbucks profiteering in the high billions. The welfare state is giving up on people like Richard. Here's my question now that it is 2010, with an election looming in the spring: do the People, the people who vote, the silent majority, do they care about the Richards of this world any more?

And then couple of months later I had to go to prison. There was a man there with diabetes, an inmate, and I was told his control was bad. Could I see him?

I caught the train over to Lewes and looked out the window at the softly rolling green hills of Sussex. What exactly went on out there in those chalky dales apart from the occasional burning of papier-mâché Popes? I'd heard about the artist Eric Gill, who once lived in Ditchling: Gill with his lovely drawings and innovative fonts. But the flip side was the shocking and criminally abusive life he led. I walked up the hill to the centre of Lewes from the station, passing posh shops and the castle. Thomas Paine lived here. Paine was in America for the revolution and then, incredibly, in France for theirs. I saw his birthplace as I neared the jail.

A large warder let me in. He then promptly locked the enormous door I'd just come through with a large key amongst a huge jingling batch that dangled from his hip. He performed this action another six times on our journey into the interior. Six doors opened and six locked behind us. I was now six solidly locked doors from the outside world, the world of those real freedoms as imagined by Thomas Paine.

The ill man was led into a stark cream-white clinical room. He was sullen, not given to japery. The reason his diabetes control was poor was simple enough to grasp: the prison diet was awful. If you wanted to reduce the prison population by encouraging atherogenesis, heart attacks and strokes amongst its inmates then his diet was the right way to go about it. Crisps, Coca-Cola, sweets: that's all our wasted prisoner lived on. Getting blood-testing strips in jail was a nightmare; something about HIV risk was mentioned. Was this institutional neglect?

I would see and hear similar stories as the years passed, hear them again and again, from nursing homes, elderly care hospitals and then, depressingly, from our own general wards. All this happened as government economic policies labelled as 'austerity measures' took hold. I saw patients who looked as if they'd been teleported from the nineteenth century. I'd say to the students and my registrars: 'That last patient looked like something out of Dickens, out of Dostoevsky.' Tatterdemalions, the near-scurvied, the near-rachitic. I'd see corkscrew hairs on the shins of some unfortunate patient and ask for vitamin C levels. Corkscrew hairs: a sign of scurvy. Nearly everyone over seventy was low in vitamin D.

This was not 1945. We had not just emerged from six years of Nazi madness, bombing and destruction. The country was clearly *very* wealthy, as evidenced by all those poncey shops on Lewes high street selling expensive tat. A high street lined with enormous people carriers not 200 yards from the clinical room in the jail. Those in power did not want to spend money on those in trouble. And the NHS itself was being undermined at all turns, spun against by the media, underfunded and undervalued. Inevitably people were getting angry. But now they were becoming angry at *us*. Shoot the messenger.

I did what I could for the prisoner and refrained from asking how long he was in for and what had he done. The warder came back for me after half an hour and then he walked me through those doors again that he locked and unlocked: 'Bad bastard, that one.'

These were his only words to me as he found the largest key for the last door. Finally, I was free. I stepped over the wooden lower frame of the exit, just like those classic scenes from a Hollywood crime caper movie: release, blessed release, into freedom. Freedom into the bright light of a beautiful sunny day in Lewes: a day that inmate I'd just seen would probably never see. Those large houses across the road from the jail, the Tudorbethan mansions, seemed incongruous, as if placed with cruel deliberation opposite the prison gates to highlight the disparity in opportunity, in fate. The elastic in the social fabric of the south-east was being stretched. Some day it might snap.

Malcolm is fretting about money and what it might buy him. He invites me to Silverstone. Malcolm is the Formula One neurosurgeon and he knows I'm trying to write a novel about a racing driver. Initially I thought of writing something about the NHS. I wanted to write about conflicting interests: the sense one had of an increasing ungratefulness and anger. An ungratefulness from a growing minority, that section of society that NHS managers insisted on calling 'clients', those who viewed medicine as a consumer product. Those who had high, and unreasonable, demands in the face of existential threats like pandemics, environmental collapse, the social and health needs of the elderly: this despite the fact that the service remained free at the point of delivery in Britain. But I was still working and it felt too close to write about what I had to do day in, day out. I was well aware of the irony of heading to Silverstone but saw it as research; how people who write defend every action.

I wanted to create a Timon of Athens figure. I wanted to invent someone disappointed by a sense of rejection now that the money had all gone, a failing team boss who had gone missing perhaps. In truth I was trying to avoid turning into a deranged version of Timon myself and thought that trying to create such a character might inoculate me, might prevent me from descending into an updated version of his despair. I was at risk of turning into one of those falling figures, the damned, in that picture Danvers and the team got me when I left Glasgow, diving down into the pit. So I displaced the action. The lead character would be a racing driver whose run of success had dried up. Malcolm was kind to help with his offer.

I dine the night before the Grand Prix with the medical team somewhere in rural Northamptonshire, the sort of place premium bond winners always seem to come from. The team are a self-satisfied lot who clearly live for cars: they are petrol-heads and have something of the rebarbative smugness that is often associated with the TV presenter Jeremy Clarkson. I should be grateful, I know, but I find myself drowning when the conversation revolves around tyre choice (Bridgestone or Pirelli), slicks versus grooves, tyre widths.

The next morning finds us in the centre of the racing circuit where there is, effectively, a small hospital: a space the size of an A+E department. I'm given the tour: there's (amazingly) a CT scanner, operative rooms, a burns unit. All geared up to deal with major trauma, subdural haematomas, you name it. The doctors wear one-piece scrubs coloured a Merlot red. They have their duties written in white capitals on their backs: ANAESTHETIST, SURGEON and so on. Another group of non-medically qualified individuals have EXTRICATOR written on their backs. Scary. There are a lot of doctors and one could, not unreasonably, argue *too* many. Who's paying for this? I'm not quite sure why Formula One needs a cardiologist on-site: the drivers have, I'm sure, fairly healthy-looking coronary arteries. I guess the cardiologists hang around to advise just in case an extricated driver has a cardiac arrest. But maybe they are there because being a doc on the Formula One circuit is very cool.

There is no one wearing the word PATHOLOGIST on his or her back. And no ENDOCRINOLOGIST either. I'm in jeans and a T-shirt but I can't help feeling that I'm a (very) small part of the team. If someone does come in hurt and they happen to have any coincidental medical condition, I might just get asked about it. I'm daydreaming: I'm a bit bored.

Helicopters are everywhere in the skies and I watch as they slowly glide in to land like giant geese. I'm reminded of images of Khe Sanh and those famous Wagner-soundtracked sequences from *Apocalypse Now*. I ask Malcolm if he knows what this airborne assault is all about and he's quick to reply: 'Oh, that's the rich arriving.' Maybe that's another reason we need the cardiologists. The race starts and I'm impressed at the level of noise. You can't get a grip on who is in the lead without glancing at the massive TV screens that make some sense of it all. The commentator jibbers on about tyres again, super-softs and dry weather compounds. I'll know more about tyres than hormones at this rate. I can hear a London colleague whispering: *That wouldn't be hard.* It's a warm day today, no sign of rain.

I take a break as the last lap approaches and sit outside the casualty unit. No one has crashed. I scan the crowds as they begin to wander back to the car parks. And then I see an obstetrician I used to work with. He's wearing an expensive Savile Row striped suit. I remember him as being something of a dandy. I could imagine him at Ascot perhaps, accompanying ladies with large hats, but here? What's he doing at a Formula One race? Standing outside the makeshift A+E I shout over to him: 'Hey, are you the on-call obstetrician? We need your help right now. We've got a delivery in here. A breech!'

He looks up in panic then recognises me and laughs. We chat, his accent still betraying his modest origins despite his best efforts to make it sound patrician, moneyed. He's here courtesy of Big Pharma. I may be wrong about the name of the company: 'Oh, I'm here courtesy of Astrastube. Got to get back to the chopper for the return flight!'

Malcolm drives me home and he makes a confession. He wants something. He wants something badly. But he's not sure if he should say. He knows it will sound bad: 'I want a Porsche.'

I nod in sympathy.

'Wouldn't we all?'

'No, you don't get it. I really want one. I've seen the one I want. I'm going to buy it. Do you think that's all right?'

I'm being asked if I can give this decision my ethical approval. Malcolm is aware that this is a luxury, that this is an indulgence that he can be criticised for succumbing to, that this is a cliché of the wealthy, the prestigious purchase that signals: *I've arrived.* I think he's asking me for my approval because he knows I come from Glasgow, he knows something of the city's history. He's asking: what would the grandson of a Glaswegian miner think of me wanting to buy a Porsche?

I'm pondering this as he speeds down the M40: is it really all right for him to buy one? He has worked hard for it. He saves lives. The billionaires who run Formula One obviously think highly enough of him to ask for his neurosurgical services. 'Well...' I hesitate and go on: 'Will it make you happy?'

He grips the wheel and takes his eyes off the road to say emphatically: 'Yes. Yes, it would. Very much.'

He says this with such emotion it's as if the Porsche is a cure for some inner angst. I'm firm: 'Then get it.'

'Are you sure?' and then, quickly, without waiting for me to reply, he adds: 'Yes, I will. I WILL.'

I prattle on about how some people go on expensive holidays to keep themselves happy; some smoke or drink, sleep around or party hard. And some, like me, buy the (very occasional) picture. He's incredulous: 'You buy art?'

'Rarely. Nothing too expensive. A few prints. It keeps me happy.'

I see him smiling. He has been absolved. His car-phone goes off and it's his wife. They chat for a bit about their kids and then he tells her: 'Baby, I've made up my mind. I'm buying the Porsche.'

I feel oddly guilty the rest of the trip home.

In my mid-twenties, around 1986 or so, I realised how deeply boring I was. I knew this beforehand, of course, since I was ten years old at least, when I understood I would never compose like Mozart or race Formula One cars or dangle from choppers or shoot Fascists. But by 1986 I knew that I needed to learn something about life outside of medicine. You can't talk about diseases every time you go on a night out with people. Diseases are a turn-off.

And so I developed a near-unhealthy interest in the life and works of Vladimir Nabokov. Why Nabokov? I got a hold of *Speak, Memory* and it seemed, to an impressionable 25-year-old, by some way the best book I'd ever read. I went through the rest of his work. I loved the jazzy Richard Lindner covers on the Penguin paperbacks. Then I wrote a couple of articles about Nabokov and medicine. I wangled a trip to Nice for an international conference where I met his son, Dmitri, and his biographer, the New Zealander Brian Boyd.

And this too: a friend for life in Pavel Dominik, Nabokov's Czech translator. I would return to Prague (after that crazy Becherovka conference) to see him many times. We would laugh together at the daffy pedantry of a few other Nabokov scholars. I wasn't immune to the madness: in Nice I did a ploddingly contrived talk on neurology as it features in Nabokov's work.

Afterwards Dmitri politely told me he enjoyed the lecture. This was a thrill, but later, over drinks with the other speakers, he threw me by asking my medical opinion: what did I think was the cause of his father's death? I had an idea but knew it would be impossible to explain succinctly. I thought that Vladimir's terminal hyponatraemia, his persistently severe low sodium, might have been due to inappropriate anti-diuretic hormone made by a bronchial cancer. Thankfully the conversation was interrupted, but then, on learning that I worked in Brighton and cared for patients with HIV with endocrine disorders, he asked me: could VN have had the virus?

Eh? Dmitri looked at me sternly, quizzically, like a college examiner looking for a fail. He was probing my professionalism, testing if I might be a crazed academic on the hunt for a scoop. I looked doubtful and shook my head in reply. Dmitri grinned in return. A wind-up, then: that famed Nabokovian laughter in the dark.

A man called Simon Karlinsky, an elderly academic who had

edited Nabokov's correspondence with Edmund Wilson, came up to me at the end of my presentation. He was way too kind and said one of the nicest things anyone, apart from my wife, has ever said to me. Karlinsky, an expert in Chekhov studies, told me: 'Anton would have loved that.'

Anton! How could he know this? He never actually *knew* Chekhov, even if he had read everything by him and about him. But Karlinsky *had* known Nabokov: he was *his* friend so maybe Simon's praise had a smidgen of validity. Maybe, just maybe, Anton (the man himself!) might just have liked my talk. Quite ludicrously I soon read minor details of Chekhov's life (and Nabokov's for that matter) and compared them to mine. In retrospect this embarrassing fact is enough of a reason for me to have sought psychiatric help.

Time to square up to The Master:

Chekhov qualified as a doctor ninety-nine years before me, in 1884. He visited Hong Kong, Singapore and Sri Lanka. I've visited Chile, Australia and Japan. He published over a hundred short stories and all those great plays. I haven't published any.

But wait, hang on: hear me out. Even if he saw patients right up to his death, by my calculations he worked as a doctor for a maximum of twenty years. Tops. I'll double-check on that. And I've done thirty-three years. I've out-doctored Chekhov by thirteen years. Beat you with that, Anton. Can we call that one-all? A score draw?

Thinking on this gives me a completely delusional sense of... what? Pride? No, not pride... It gives me a crazy sense of... victory. I make it 2–1 in extra time. Chekhov might have posthumous fame, he might be a literary genius, but I've out-doctored him. I've seen more patients than Chekhov. *Soooperb.*

I know, I know. I could have done a few more years, done more doctoring. Maybe I *should* have gone on to do the full forty. By then

I'd be sixty-two; my dad died when he was sixty-two. I think Anton died at an age when he was still occasionally seeing patients. So I have to face it, the actual final score is a trouncing: 100 or more published short stories to nil.

How did he get the time to write so much? But then people bug me who say: how do you get the time to read so much? When I recommend a recently published novel, this is what I am sometimes asked. Translated this means: *You're a real lazy bastard, aren't you?* And they are right, of course. I really should have been reading the latest paper on IGFBP-5 at two in the morning, but I'm boring enough as it is. I was boring *myself*.

I can't help concluding Chekhov couldn't have seen *that* many patients, not really. He made his quip about medicine being his lawful wife and writing his mistress, but I don't see him as being the most uxorious of men. I think he was off scribbling with that floozy and attending the sick only when he was up for it: that, and his worrying all night about chasing rabbits. And then you have to factor in the days he must have been off sick with TB.

It's a good excuse for a day off, TB. I can picture him giving his excuses to some manager, some Russian ogre: 'I can't do the clinic today, boss, because – cough, cough – I'm chucking up blood, I'm having a haemoptysis as we speak. It's my TB playing up again.' Staring down into his blood-stained hanky.

I took no more than thirty days off in thirty-three years, if that, because of annual doses of the flu before the vaccine. That and one other prolonged event we will come to. One vascular surgeon I know nearing sixty tells me he hasn't taken a single day off sick. Not one.

Pre-Covid-19, doctors loaded with the flu, still hacking and spluttering, would go back in, nose streaming, eyes stinging. Many forced themselves to return because the clinics would get overbooked and you were made to feel that you were just making life difficult for yourself and your patients if you didn't turn up. It was just another way the underfunding of the NHS fucked everyone over. This would come back to haunt us big style.

But what about TB? If you went down with the Chekhov's, that meant you would be off on the sick for an age. TB meant 'get a locum'.

When I was a medical student we were once taken to a place that looked after the young chronically sick. Many of these places were closed down in the early Thatcher years. Unfortunate people who had sustained a serious brain injury after a motorcycle accident might end up here; ditto those with rheumatic heart disease (people similar to my Aunt June) who were unlucky enough to have had a stroke after a clot flipped up to the brain as a result of a faulty heart valve.

There was one room I'll never forget where maybe twenty young people were propped up against the walls. This was a group of tragic individuals born with severe learning difficulties, often all-too-casually, insensitively, labelled as 'syndromic'. One of them lifted his hands as we were escorted past. His fingers were fused into a giant lobster-like claw. Another had hydrocephalus, with his characteristic large skull. Those cruel voices from my childhood piped up as they watched from the touchline: *Heid! Heid that baw!* Another man-child pirouetted incessantly, a kid born with a critical loss of oxygen to the brain. Outside, the late afternoon sun lit the green-brown Campsie Fells. More fortunate people were out on the mountains climbing, walking.

The place was called after a castle and I couldn't help but be reminded of the Nazis and their euthanasia Aktion T4 madness. These people I was looking at in the castle were similar to the people who suffered under Hitler. Tiergartenstrasse 4 was the address in Berlin where 'plans' were made for the chronically sick, the economically 'unviable'. Those atrocities occurred in out-of-the-way places, out in the country. Unseen, unheard. 'Euthanasia', they called it. But the Nazis knew they were murdering them.

I doubted my skills looking after those with learning difficulties, thinking I lacked the patience to care for them properly, thinking I'd be paralysed by pity, but my actual experiences working with them were revelatory. It struck me on more than one occasion that some had been blessed with an inner vision. Some had a way of seeing things like a child, an innocence that stripped away many of the delusions the so-called 'normal' majority entertain. Oliver Sacks describes how a few stroke patients with a receptive dysphasia (an inability to understand language) would often laugh uproariously at politicians on the TV because they understood from the vocal tone *alone* that they, and we, were being lied to.

I regularly saw one young lady born with microcephaly, a small brain, a condition back in the news recently after the Zika virus outbreak in Brazil. She was small in height too and her parents dressed her neatly like the little girl she really was. She was in her early forties; her parents in their sixties. When I spoke to her she would smile and sometimes cover her face shyly. And when I would say something to her that might come across as condescending, as for example: 'Do you like music?', she would look up and say cheekily: 'Shut up.' This came out like this: *Shuh hup*. Banter. Her voice a gentle, high-pitched wind-up that meant: *Careful, you're at risk of boring me.* Her parents would gently remonstrate with her, but I loved it. She had an unerring sense for bullshit, or so it seemed. And she would giggle when she said it again after I asked her another lame question: 'Is that a new doll you've got?'

'Shuh hup.'

'Do you like watching the TV?'

'Shuh hup.'

'Do you like cartoons?'

Louder now. 'SHUH HUP!' And then she gets the giggles again.

With other patients who have learning difficulties I might ask about what they were doing later on that day, what was happening this coming summer, were they going away anywhere? I'd find out from the men which football team they supported; this was hugely helpful. Each time I'd see them we would talk about the ups and downs of their team. Getting trust was essential and given the time pressures, identifying what it was that *really* interested them was a crucial way of making contact. You've got to try and break out of your own interiority, the limits of your own mental cell, be open to what drives others. Try to escape the fate of Nabokov's famous trapped ape, his image of a limited consciousness: an ape drawing the bars of its cage.

14

A FREE TRIP TO SYDNEY

Here's another young woman with diabetes who keeps being admitted with ketoacidosis. She's nearly died on several occasions. She tells us that her diabetes is 'brittle' and that it isn't her fault. 'Brittle' diabetes is a much-debated label. Most clinicians think that people are (*de facto*) brittle; they do not have 'brittle' diabetes per se. Her angry insistence on her having 'brittle' diabetes convinces me that she is herself, in some way, the solution. She isn't taking her insulin. It's my job to get her to admit this to herself and for her to confront the issue head on. I sit at her bedside: 'Do you know why this is happening?'

'Well, yes. My diabetes is just brittle, that's all. There must be something odd about it.'

'Yes, there is something odd about it. What do you think that might be?'

'I don't know. Maybe my body doesn't respond to insulin or something.'

'That's very rare. That's really very unusual. And because you have told me you sometimes get hypos, low blood sugars, I know that your body can definitely respond to insulin.'

'So, what's wrong with me then?'

'I think maybe you can help me answer that. I think you know the answer to that question.'

'I don't.'

She's very insistent. She has said something similar every time she has been admitted over these past fifty occasions. Fifty admissions to hospital in five years. Maybe an average stay of four days. So 200 days in hospital. I can hear one of our managers quoting the cost of an average day's stay in hospital. Two hundred days of her short life have seen her cooped up here with the incontinent, the delirious, a few ranting junkies and some verbally abusive alcoholics. Her frustration is now spilling over. She's angry and she's close to shouting at me. I try again, leaning in, talking in a quieter, gentler tone: 'Can I tell you what I *think* is going on?'

Hesitantly she answers: 'Yes, you can try.'

'I think maybe, just maybe, that you sometimes forget to take your insulin.'

'No, NO! Never! I *always* take it, always!'

I drop my voice, now almost a whisper: 'OK. Now let's go slowly, listen to me please. I know *why* you don't want to tell me that you miss it.'

'I don't. I never miss it!'

'Hang on.'

'I never miss it. Are you calling me a liar?'

Her aggressive responses are telling us both the truth: 'No, I'm not. Not at all. Listen. It can be very hard to admit to something. I know you think that we would be unhappy with you if you were missing injections. But listen carefully: we're not your parents. We're not your teachers. We're not the police. We are *not* going to get you into trouble. This is about getting you *out* of trouble. You are already at real risk of harming yourself. We are not going to shout at you or lecture you. We're not going to judge you.'

'YOU ARE!'

She starts to sob quietly. I try again: 'I'm not. We're not. Look… I – we – only want to help you. We're not going to condemn you or shout at you or whatever. I only want to see you get better. If you tell me that you have missed your insulin then fine, I can understand that. Who would want to jab themselves daily anyway? That must be awful.'

I've hit a nerve.

'It is.'

'I know it is. I've done it once or twice myself when I've been teaching, shown the students what an injection is like, and I didn't like it. Admitting that to yourself is the first thing to do. Admitting your fear. We can understand that. And we can help you with it. There's plenty of things *I'm* scared of.'

'You won't be angry with me?'

'No, I promise. Of course I won't.'

She has lived in fear of anger all her life. Lived in fear of her elders castigating her for not doing what they have told her to do. Her rebellion pains her. She murmurs 'OK' and leans over her bed to pull up a bag she has stashed underneath. She opens it slowly. Inside are about 100 unopened little glass bottles of insulin.

She starts to cry very hard. I give her time and then say: 'That's OK. That's OK. Steady. We'll sort this out for you. Don't worry. You've done the right thing.'

She looks up imploringly: 'Have I?'

This is what Rosamund Bartlett says about Chekhov in her introduction to his letters: 'With some justification he also feared that his professional reputation as a doctor might be jeopardised if people knew about his alter ego as a humorous writer for lowbrow journals.'

Chekhov also knew he wasn't a fuckin' comedian.

Bartlett reports a detail as she studies Chekhov's notations: 'His handwriting became smaller and smaller.' Reading this, I laugh out loud in recognition. My own micrographic scrawl has been called out many times. As a consultant it even cropped up in one of my appraisals: *Your writing can be... tiny, difficult to read.*

Can you imagine someone doing an appraisal of Chekhov? Imagine a colleague saying this to the great man, aged around forty: 'Well, we like what you do, Anton, you're great but... could you maybe write a little bit larger?'

One senior colleague, a saturnine fellow who didn't mince his words, challenged me when I was a registrar: 'Your writing is minuscule. You must have an anal personality.'

I met him years later at a college party with Cycling Scott. Scott greeted him with: 'Are you still as much of a fascist as ever?' To which he answered: 'Of course!'

Bartlett makes me smile again, this time ruefully, when I read that Chekhov, an ardent Dreyfusard, fell out with the publisher Aleksey Suvorin over the anti-Semitism of the latter's newspaper. I grin sadly because I haven't seen one friend since a discussion we had about the Middle East. He was (and still is, I assume) passionately pro-Palestinian. We were dining with our wives in an Italian restaurant. Wine had flowed. The 2014 referendum on Scottish independence was looming and he asked how we planned to vote. I explained that as English residents we didn't have a vote, which is as it should be. 'But if you were allowed to, how would you vote: not for independence, surely?'

This asked in a sceptical tone, his BBC RP accent hinting that he would consider a vote for secession rank betrayal. I slightly resent his presumption, his encoded post-imperialist superiority. Megalo-thymia. *You couldn't possibly want to split from us. After all we've done for you.* I'm riled but try to surprise him with: 'Well, it just so happens that I got a phone call last week from Nicola. You know Nicola, don't you?'

It's my turn to be condescending. He's aghast: 'What! That woman with the ridiculous haircut? Your so-called First Minister? Wee Jimmy Krankie herself? Sturgeon? C'mon, you're joking, right?'

'No, I'm not. She had a job offer for me.'

'You what?'

'Yes, well, she's having to consider who she should appoint to var-ious ambassadorial roles in a future independent Scotland.'

'Oh yeah! And?'

His voice is now raised, he's indignant and he's not hiding it very well. I explain: 'Well, Nicola called me and said that she had been made aware by others of my love for Joseph Roth (ridiculously I pronounce this, properly of course, as *Yosep Rote*) and Philip Roth (pronounced Philip Roth) and Walter Benjamin (again, without laughing, I say *Valter Benyahmeen*) and Norman Mailer and so, well, would I like to be Edinburgh's first ambassador to Israel? Would I like to relocate to Tel Aviv?'

His mouth is open and then he gasps: 'You haven't said yes, have you?'

'Of course I have! Tel Aviv will be great. All that Bauhaus archi-tecture, the beach, the nightlife.'

He's strident now. He's incandescent: 'You FUCKER! How could you?'

His partner is rocking with laughter, but he is not amused. There's no coming back from that and not long after we leave the restaurant.

As said, I haven't seen him since. Another practical joke that failed. Another pratfall: another reminder that I'm not a fuckin' whatever.

In my mid-forties I accept a job at the Deanery: an associate dean post based in London, on Tooley Street to be exact, not far from London Bridge Station. The commute from Brighton would be straightforward. This part of the city was being transformed fast. The new mayor's office resembled a giant silver testicle and there were plans to build a gigantic shard of glass, a skyscraper straight out of Bruno Taut's more outlandish dreams. I'd work there every Friday and get a day away from the endless clinical pressures, the remorseless freneticism of activity on the wards. Like many before me, I needed a bit of a break.

The team up at the Deanery was friendly and very London in manner: quick-witted, gossipy but focused, prone to long, albeit productive, lunches. The new Dean had honed organisation skills and set me to work on those trainees thought to be troubled: the so-called 'trainees in difficulty', or TIDs. We reckoned that around 5 per cent of our postgraduates were struggling. This 5 per cent we could break down further. One third of them were unwell: this was something we could deal with; we could point them towards those who could care for them best. We were doctors, after all, and if we could not deal with our own then who could? But it was not always easy to identify sickness. A doctor could, for example, be branded as being easily distracted or lazy and then only later be found to have a brain tumour. We often asked a tame neurologist to review a TID to ensure we were not missing out on any occult organic pathology. Or we'd call in a psychiatrist. One of my key reasons for joining the Deanery was to try to prevent situations like Jim, that guy who shot himself when I was an SHO. I had felt for years since his death that no one was really looking out for him. Maybe I was wrong, but any prophylactic measures to avoid a repetition seemed worthwhile.

Another third of TIDs were struggling because of system failures: they were in the wrong unit for training or overburdened with shift work or whatever. This too was a situation that we at the Deanery could quickly and easily resolve.

But it was the final third, that 1.5 per cent of trainees, who caused us the most heartache, the greatest angst. These were trainees with no insight: the sociopaths. I recall one guy who was taking an inordinately long time to finish training. He was in his forties, technically still a junior, and when we first met he rejected the criticisms levelled at him by his educational supervisor. His supervisor was a senior colleague, one of the most respected opinions in the country, and his central critique of the trainee revolved around availability; doesn't it always? The bosses couldn't find this trainee when he was most needed.

We decided to settle the matter by allocating no fewer than *four* separate educational supervisors to him for his next post at a major London teaching hospital. These supervisors were no fools. They knew our suspicions. There was talk that he was moonlighting at another hospital. Eight months later we meet up with him again and have all four of the educational supervisors' reports. Each accuses him of not answering bleeps, of absenteeism. Again there is the concern that he has been heading to another hospital at the weekends to earn money, only to then arrive late on Monday mornings. I put this accusation to him and he answers: 'No, that's not correct.'

He's adamant that he is always available. I press on, hoping that I appear calm: 'So, are you saying that all four of these respected colleagues of ours are lying in their reports?'

'No, I'm not saying that.'

'Well, I put it to you that all four of these doctors say that you are rarely around, that they can never seem to get a hold of you when you are paged.'

It was difficult (a) not to lose the rag with him and (b) not to come over like a cross-examining barrister: *I put it to you*. And yet, as I speak with him, I'm constantly aware that I must not appear to be harassing. Or bullying. We have policies for that too. He could accuse *us*. We could lose *our* jobs. Such is the face, the tragi-comic farce, of the modern NHS. This is the difficulty we have in holding people to account.

We reach an impasse, the usual he said/she said stuff. Eventually it is decided that he will be seconded to another Deanery for yet another fresh team of assessors.

I work with more complex cases. Doctors with Asperger's, doctors with schizophrenia. We try to keep the TIDs working, but it is sometimes clear that the chances of them becoming a consultant are low. Their record of absenteeism is just too extensive and inconsistent to ensure proper training. And yet legally it is very difficult to terminate a doctor from training, short of them being suspended by the GMC. This can be very frustrating when you know they are taking up a training post that is much coveted by other highly capable individuals. Perhaps another career choice will be a more practical option, a more beneficial and happier path for them to take.

I try to acquire diplomatic skills, learn how to chair meetings, understand the jargon of feedback, encourage best practice. Progress is often glacial. We visit hospitals on inspections. I get to know the layout of many hospitals, which one does a decent breakfast, which one has horrendous parking. Meetings drag on into the early evening. There are more wash-up sessions. The Dean signals he's had enough by blowing his nose into his handkerchief, his blasts proudly thunderous.

Inwardly I giggle at a senior GP, an exile from Khomeini's Iran, whose accent (who am I to laugh at others' accents?) persistently renders another colleague's name 'Graeme' as 'Gram'. Every time he calls him Gram I have vision of country rock star Gram Parsons and those brilliantly wild white suits he once wore: Nudie jackets with their designs featuring lurid crucifixes and sacred hearts. Gram with his C+W tunes, slide geetars a-twanging. Graeme is nothing like Gram: he's from Chichester and doesn't have a Nudie jacket. Not that I'm aware of.

A couple of months later and, after a flight, I'm at an evening team-building meeting with managers in another part of the UK. I'm listening to the key speaker, an academic leader. Her talk is hot on references to inclusivity. She goes into battle wearing her knowledge of Foucault like a shield and enjoys bamboozling others with quotations from Chomsky or Derrida or Barthes. She correctly pronounces the latter as 'Bart' and I see some of the others thinking: What the hell has *The Simpsons* got to do with plans for regional reconfiguration of services? She digs interdisciplinary studies. I meet her after I've done a morning clinic at my own hospital and she asks me how my day has been so far. I answer: 'I saw a few transgender patients.'

'Oh, yes?'

'Yes, and I was thinking whether I should tell them that they were looking more feminine, or masculine, you know... comment on their appearance.'

'Uh huh.'

She's looking at me quizzically and (am I imagining this?) with more than a hint of scorn. I press on naïvely: 'You don't think saying something like that is a good idea then?'

She's curt: 'No.'

And then turns on her heels.

Much later I tell the story to a colleague who works at this hospital and, to my surprise, he falls about laughing at my mistake. He tells me that she's an expert and has supervised PhD theses on the impact of gender reassignment.

Getting the identifier, the pronoun, right is all-important when dealing with trans patients. Some prefer to be referred to in a neutral manner: 'I saw Ally at the clinic today. They are feeling well at present.' Always ask which pronoun they prefer. *They*. Trans patients get enough hassle from the general public and social media without you exacerbating the challenges they face. Every time I read some commentator from either the right or the left on TV being dismissive or trivial about trans people (and their right to healthcare) I find myself wishing I could teleport said talking head to my clinic and then tell them: *OK, you take over now, say what you just said on TV to this person, right here, right now.*

This is particularly true of patients with the syndrome called testicular feminisation. In this condition people are born XY (i.e. genetically male) but are insensitive to testosterone: testosterone as a key does not work with their testosterone receptors as a lock. Phenotypically they look female. They are brought up female: they *are* female. I'd like to know what Germaine Greer and other vocal polemicists think about testicular feminisation. Here's the *hing*, as we say in Glasgow: you don't know what someone's cells are up to by just looking at their face. You know nothing of their chromosomes or their hormones or their receptors by just meeting them. *At's the hing.*

Care; do no harm; be sensitive; *think*. One of my registrars was threatened with legal proceedings after filling in a blood request form. Under the section asking the reason for the test the registrar had written 'gender dysphoria'. The patient complained because they rejected this terminology. As far as they were concerned, they had no dysphoria: they were who they were. There was no *dys-* about it. The registrar duly apologised: they were in a hurry and due down in A+E; eight new patients were waiting to be seen, they had scribbled the request too fast. The threat was politely withdrawn.

Later still I write a glowing review of Jeffrey Eugenides's book *Middlesex* for the *British Medical Journal* and not long after get a call from a person with 5-alpha-reductase deficiency. This is the syndrome featured in the novel in which a young person raised as a girl undergoes male changes at puberty. I meet with this extraordinary human, this brave person who has faced unknowable levels of prejudice.

Our first conversation, rightly, fittingly given our introduction, is about language; *Middlesex* has mightily impressed them too. What we need to be clear about right from the off is what pronoun we need to use. They want to use 'they'. Not he, not she and, God forbid, never, ever, ever *it*. Too many people for far too long have treated trans people as an 'it'. They, my patient, see themself as 'post-gender'. They see themself, rightly, as special. They have a lot to tell us, to instruct us. They can teach us about constructs of gender, about bigotry, about premature judgements based on surface appearance.

Not for the first time as an endocrinologist I find myself trying to get my head around the awfulness of being a person who has undergone multiple genital operations as a child. The sheer horror of this: and I'm struck at the clinic by how many of these traumatised people, some of the best people, the best humans I've ever met, how many have somehow retained a faith in humanity despite all their suffering. Somehow they retain patience with the ignorant. They burn with a need to instruct, to enlighten, to correct, to ask quietly yet insistently that they be treated as equals with the rest of us. They never asked for this to happen to them and they need, they demand, our support.

After I pass my fiftieth birthday I note an advertisement in the *British Medical Journal* for a Dean's post in Sydney. I've never been to Australia and until now have had little interest in going. But, what the heck, it's a quiet weekend at home so I've time to fill out the forms for a laugh.

Oz, Aussies. What do I know of the place? Not much. I've long hated Rolf Harris and once threw a record of his out a window from a flat we were renting on Hove seafront. The song had a cringe-inducing title: 'Someone's Pinched Me Winkles'. I watched the disc skite over an empty dual carriageway to land intact on a pitch and putt course. Did I rate anything from Down Under? I had a long-standing attraction to the music of the Go-Betweens and (our near-neighbour!) Nick Cave. I'm indifferent to kangaroos, koalas. Australia was not first on the list as a site for a new life.

We had a Skype chat first and then, to my surprise, they invited me over for a formal interview. I was told they would pay for the flights and a week's stay in a central Sydney hotel. 'Oh, and your wife can come over too, of course.' Hey... a week's free holiday in Australia!

I talked with our chief executive. I wanted his advice: would he back such a move?

'Sure. 100 per cent. Go for it, John.'

'I'm just a bit worried that if I got it and then didn't really like it I'd...'

'No worries. I'll make sure you are on secondment. For up to five years if you like.'

Wow, five years! This was a ludicrously generous offer. Could he truly authorise such an arrangement? As CE he had previously been supportive with challenges facing our specialty. I'd seen him in action at board meetings: he didn't refrain from giving robust critique of failing projects. He wasn't a fuckin' comedian either. One time I met him in the car park chatting to a guy who looked like a Thunderbird pilot and he asked me how everything was going. Inside I'm raging and told him straight that things were shite. There were no beds and it was a fucking disaster. He gestured to the man and said: 'John, meet the Secretary of State, Andy Burnham.'

And so we flew out. A cab was waiting for us at the airport. The driver had a Greek name; this didn't surprise me. I knew there were more Athenians in Australia than in Athens or some such. His xenophobic rant on the drive into town alarmed me; he was angry with immigrants. Given that I'd been in the country a mere hour I didn't think it politic to point out that surely he was one too. Wasn't his type of attitude, on the rise in Britain too, one of the things I wanted to escape from?

He dropped us off at the hotel near the main railway station. We dumped our bags and then, jet-lagged, walked downtown like zombies to hit the harbour and catch a boat out to Manly. Sydney was as lovely as Jan Morris said it would be in her fantastic book that I'd read on the flight over. And then we were on the Corso and awed by the beach: one of the most stunning on the planet. We were beginning to get the point of Australia.

I admired the cosmopolitan nature of the crowd. These were ordinary people carrying surfboards and swimming gear, not the tanned gods we were used to seeing on the imported soaps on British TV.

These families were not poor, but they weren't rich either; they were the great middle. We admired the scallop forms of the Opera House on the way back and ate well on seafood in a restaurant near The Rocks. The great iron coat hanger-shaped bridge nearby stretched over the calm waters, the yachts.

I did a presentation to the faculty and chose to talk about failure and what we can learn from it, how central failure is to progress. I used the over-familiar Sam Beckett exhortation: fail better and all that yackety-yak. I think the talk went down OK; I got a few laughs. Later my wife and I walked around Darlinghurst and Paddington checking out the properties. These were out-of-our-reach expensive to buy, but we would be renting if I got the job. One day we crossed the waters to Balmain and ate bugs (the large crayfish they seem to major in over there) and admired sandstone villas lined with exotic plants. Sydney had a smell and it was wonderful: cool eucalyptus and hot jacaranda. I'd never been in a city so floral, so pleasing to the olfactory sense. The unusual bird life was fascinating. Strange creatures strutted and ate from the bins: trash turkeys; noisy miners and sulphur-crested cockatoos hopping at a bus stop; rainbow-coloured lorikeets perched on the electric wires strung across the streets. And a kookaburra chuckled somewhere high up a gum. We sang that song we learned at school: *Merry merry king of the bush is he / laugh, kookaburra, laugh.*

The time for the interview had arrived. I walked through the halls of the new medical school and saw... crucifixes. This was a single-faith medical school: a Catholic medical school. What was I doing here? I hadn't been to confession for years. What if I'm rumbled? Well, if that happened, as John Lennon once sang: they're gonna crucify me.

I'm introduced to the panel. There is no medical presence. The

Dean of Jurisprudence is here and the Dean of Divinity, who kicks off the show. He speaks in an accent (as my pal Danvers would surely note) like the mythical Lance Ritchie: 'Good morning, John, and thank you for coming all this way.'

He pronounces 'way' as 'why'.

'I'd like to begin the interview. Can I ask what your views are on assisted reproduction?'

Whit?

The interview continues in this pointedly ethical vein and I say what I think I believe. There are enthusiastic nods when I state blandly that my understanding, as a doctor trained in biology, is that human life, Jim, as we know it, could be said to begin at conception. I didn't say that Jim bit. The zealous nodding of the panel leads me to conclude that they have another entirely different agenda in mind. Oh hell, they are going to ask me my thoughts on the 'right to life' controversy.

A face flashes in memory. I can see her again in my mind: my Aunt June, dead more than ten years now. June: my Catholic aunt who needed warfarin; who fell pregnant. Who was told she couldn't go to term because it would kill her. Who was told the baby would be damaged by the warfarin. I can see her again, her pleading stare that night when she had a belly full of ascitic fluid, *ass–cite–ease*, that night she was dying, that night she watched the towers fall on 9/11. Her desperate eyes asking me: *It'll be all right, won't it?*

Somehow I get through the questioning without overtly upsetting the panel, or finding myself having to lie, or saying something I do not actually believe. After, I meet up with my wife in a nearby pub. Maybe I was a plausible candidate. Maybe they might even give me the job. Jeez: if so I'll have to meet the Cardinal.

I can't see me meeting the Cardinal. Meeting the Cardinal on a regular basis. I can't imagine a discussion with the Cardinal about

Nabokov's *Ada* or George Grosz's *Ecce Homo* sketches. Maybe he'd even make me make a confession to him. See me behind the grill: bless me, Father, it's been a couple of decades since I last confessed. I've sworn, been greedy, got drunk, watched *Behind Convent Walls*.

The same pub in the early evening after the interview: some of the members of the panel have arrived. And it is here and now that I understand the *real* interview has begun. Maybe this is how they do things in Australia. One of the Deans drinks deep of his pint, wipes his unruly beard and asks in Strine: 'John, as an endocrine specialist, do you treat any of those gender-bender types?'

Those were his exact words. *Gender-bender types.* The ocker stereotype has just arrived in my face. I'm a guest in his country and try very hard to conceal my distaste for his question (why should I have to?), but when I answer forcefully – *yes, yes I do* – I know that my jolly little holiday trip to Australia is well and truly over.

My interrogators move on to domestic politics dashed with some more casual racism. Theirs is a more poisonous anti-immigrant rhetoric, if delivered with a tad more linguistic subtlety, than the Greek taxi driver's rants at the airport: they don't call new arrivals 'fuckers'.

Australia, Catholic Australia anyway, was somewhere politically to the right of contemporary Catholic Austria, the Austria excoriated by Thomas Bernhard. This was not good. It may be nice and sunny and hot and have lots of funny animals and a great smell, but Catholic Oz was a pit of reactionary old farts more at home in a rural Irish seminary. Back in England I get a call two weeks later to say that they've given the job to someone else: 'You did very well, John. And don't worry about it: the person we gave it to is a close personal friend of Julia Gillard, our PM.'

15

SHINGLES

JULY 1884, ZVENIGOROD

'I spend half the day seeing patients (thirty to forty a day) and the rest of the time I relax or bore myself horribly sitting by the window looking out at the grey skies which for three days now have been relentlessly tipping down a most disagreeable rain … In front of my window there is a hill with pine trees; to the right is the police chief's house, and further round in the same direction a scruffy little town which once was an important city…'

APRIL 2016, BRIGHTON

I spend most of the day seeing patients (thirty to forty a day) and the rest of the time I relax or bore myself pleasantly sitting by the window looking out at the grey skies which for three days now have been relentlessly tipping down a most disagreeable rain … In front of my window there is a white church that looks Greek and a small cul-de-sac that ends in some garages where two cats sit on the roof and occasionally spit and hiss at each other … I set my iPhone to YouTube and listen to an early Steely Dan demo called 'Gullywater' that reminds me of Rhoda Morgenstern and Manhattan and Manhattans…

Check, Dr Chekhov, check.

One day, after seeing another thirty patients, I'm looking out at the white Greek church opposite before completing the final email session of the day. The phone rings. Every doctor knows the heart-sink feeling on getting a call just as you are about to leave for home. You can almost taste your evening meal, then... the summons to the ward or to ITU that means arriving home a couple of hours later. Food is wasted. Wives or husbands or partners despair. Patients come first.

I pick up the phone and hear a woman's voice, one that is vaguely familiar.

'Hello?'

'Yes, hello, Dr Quin. Remember me? We met for the first time this afternoon.'

'Can you remind me please? Sorry!'

Apologising again. The eightieth apology today. I don't want to say that I've seen thirty patients earlier and can't recall all their voices.

'Yes, it's Helen. I was telling you all about my tiredness earlier.'

I remember her story quickly but only dimly visualise the lady's face: 'Ah, yes! How can I help you, Helen?'

Complaints against the NHS are on a steeply rising curve and the best approach to anyone calling up to moan is to deal with their concerns as quickly and as politely as possible. Inevitably this puts even more strain on the system. It is also personally draining. My communication skills are adequate – the result, I think, of being brought up well by my parents and attending a mixed-ability school. But the endless apologising on behalf of the system is taking its toll. All my colleagues tell me they too seem to be saying 'sorry' almost hourly. Apologising in a pleasant, non-confrontational manner to angry people who are swearing at you is... tiring. Especially when they threaten to call up the newspapers or their MP. Such bullying behaviour is generally accompanied with a whine about the state of the country or a few casual racist slurs: more xenophobic griping about immigrants. And then once a month this person will say something like this: 'Ai pie your effin' salary, y'know!'

Quite often this comes from chippier young professionals: Thatcher's children. They've had enough of *experts*. Experts, as told to them by the politicians they champion, are old hat. We've heard enough from experts.

They sit impatiently, looking at their watch as you fill in a form for them, huffing and puffing: *I've got a meeting up in London to get to, you know.* Their mantra is this: ask not what your country can do for you; ask what your country *owes* you. Their anger at almost everything is ill concealed. They want to exclude people, they want to build walls, they want, want, want. This is what I want to say to them. Indulge me. Here's my reverie: 'You pay *my* salary?'

'Yeah, you hert royt.'

'How much do you think you pay towards my salary?'

'Well, 'ow the hell should I know that?'

'You've said you pay my salary, so how much of my pay has been your *direct* contribution?'

'Look: don't get angry wif me, mate. I'm 'ere to get my money's wuff.'

'I see you work in the City.'

'What of it?'

'Well, let's say you do actually declare your tax, which I doubt, but let's give you the benefit of that not-unreasonable doubt and let's say you paid, oh, let's be generous, £40k in tax last year. I know, I know, I know that you didn't pay even a fraction of that, but let's say that you did.'

Ever the son of a tax inspector. Here I fantasise that I take out a calculator, tap in some data dividing his contribution into the active workforce numbers, and conclude: 'That means that you do indeed pay my salary. You do! How about that? You have contributed around 2p to my annual earnings in the past ten years.'

My fantastical high-flying broker is quick to come back at me: 'Fink you're fahking smart, douncha?'

And here I rummage in my pocket and pull out a bronze coin, toss it to him, and then bark in an accent redolent of one of those meth-addled refugees from the Sarry Heid pub: 'Here's your two fuckin' pee. Now on your way, pal. GET THE FUCK RIGHT OUT OF MY FUCKIN' SURGERY!'

You can take the boy out of Glasgow. An English friend once trotted out that old cliché after he listened to another of my long moans. The fact that the NHS is provided free at the point of delivery is wholly taken for granted by this minority of malcontents. They salivate over the hand they love to feed on. But, thankfully, these arseholes are less than 5 per cent of the patients we see, a percentage eerily similar to those doctors in trouble I dealt with at the Deanery. The problem they share is this: a fundamental lack of insight. Future neurobiological testing will no doubt confirm these people to be psychopaths.

To return to that surprise phone call. Helen gets back to me: 'Yes, you can help, Dr Quin. Would you like to have a cup of coffee with me?'

I do a double-take at the handset now away from my ear. What was that? Did I hear her correctly? Is this a wind-up or what?

'I...'

'There's a nice coffee shop nearby called Ground. Fancy that?'

Words are shouting in my head – NO, NO, NO, NO, NOOOO – I'M A MARRIED MAN!

'I...'

My brain wants to say it calmly: 'I'm a happily married man.' But I quickly catch myself because she's asking to meet over a cup of coffee. That's all. But wait: isn't that a date? I'm being presumptuous: surely she doesn't want to go out with me? Thinking quickly, I say: 'I… I don't think that would be appropriate, do you? I'm sorry… I hope that's OK.'

She's quick to come back; she's embarrassed, now speaking hurriedly: 'No, of course, of course. You're quite right. Sure. No worries.'

'I'll make sure to send you a copy of your clinic letter. Is there anything else I can do for you?'

'No, no, that's fine. Take care and bye-bye.'

She hangs up.

I stare at the phone. This has never happened to me in my thirty-plus-year career. I'm balding, I'm putting on weight, I'm nearing fifty. And now and only now does someone ask me out for coffee. I think carefully. I should document this. Just in case. That's the world doctors live in today. Document it. You never know what someone might say. I call the medical director, who sympathises.

I do the clinics with a medical student or a nurse in attendance and document the name of the student in my letters as I dictate in front of the patient: 'I saw Mr/Mrs/Miss Williams today along with my third-year medical student/nurse Jo/Joe.'

A witness, then: paranoid times require careful practice. One colleague undergoes a two-year investigation after an allegation of assault. I used to see him at the clinic as a patient because of his medical condition. He would always come along with his wife for support. They were suffering. I watched as their faces became ever more drained. The pressure mounted and then the case was heard. He was duly exonerated. His relief, when I next saw him, was even more evident than the time I told him his cancer was gone.

The medical director wants a favour. He asks me to investigate a complaint of harassment. I say sure but soon wish I hadn't. The complainant, 'A', is a trainee and his boss, 'B', a consultant, backs him. A says that another consultant, 'C', has been bullying him; C has been harassing him. He says that C has called him lazy or some such. A alleges that this event was not a one-off: C has been giving him a hard time. I arrange to meet all three of them separately and go through each of their stories. It quickly becomes apparent that A is not the most impressive trainee I've ever met and that he and B have met several times to discuss the issue. I cannot rule out collusion between the two. But, but, but…

I have little doubt either after meeting with C that he is overly defensive. I'm, oh, about 70 per cent sure he has been harassing A. But getting proof from another (fourth) party proves impossible. I cannot triangulate the evidence. People clam up when I ask their view of C. And then I learn why. I'm told C is litigious. I send in my report and the HR department is not happy. They want a guilty or not guilty verdict. I've gone for the Scots option: *not proven*. If I find him guilty without enough evidence, I know I'm open to legal challenge from C. That means years of pain trying to deal with this *and* (like Mr Chekhov) somehow continuing to see those thirty-plus patients on a two-clinic day.

I suspect deep down that C is not *not* guilty. The HR department put me under heavy pressure to come down on one side of the coin. I resist and insist that he be given my report which concludes that the case against him is not proven. The case is closed.

The pressures mount: money is running out for the NHS. Under-investment puts a strain on everything. Colleagues are tired, irritable; it is an effort to stay calm, stay cool. A friend has his contract terminated after he was alleged to have made unwise remarks about another trainee. He too is exonerated. It's slash and burn time in the NHS and morale is at rock-bottom. Things will only get worse.

I'm now fifty-two and an ill-defined pain in my back comes on; it lasts about four days. I'm thinking maybe I need a scan when one night, as I leap out of bed to go to the bathroom, my wife yells: 'Look at your back!' There it is, the classic red weal-like lesions of herpes zoster, the shingles. I look as if I've been whipped with jaggy nettles. I'm amazed at how painful it becomes: I'm prostrate with agony and take the first full week off sick in my career. I can't lie on the side of the blistering. I can't sleep. Now I know what hell my patients have gone through when they've had the condition.

Shingles: the word itself makes the condition sound trivial, makes you think of beaches, Brighton beach perhaps, and the soothing sound of surf on pebbles. Forget that: shingles is fucking awful. Eventually I struggle back to work and find myself at a morning handover. We sit in a large room where the night shift tells the day team what patients have come in overnight. The gang's all here: maybe fourteen or so juniors and six consultants, everyone present and correct apart from another consultant. He's late.

Then he arrives without an apology. Sometimes he struggles to accept patients who are clearly his responsibility. Another colleague chairing the handover loses patience with him: 'Listen, this patient is yours.'

'No, I don't think so. It doesn't sound significant. He should be under you.'

This silliness goes on and on. And the juniors are watching. The recalcitrant consultant is a repeat offender. I recall one weekend when he refused to see *five* patients, each of whom had an issue related to his specialty. Eventually, after pleading, he saw them.

The juniors around the table are appalled and titillated by this public disagreement between the seniors. Once they have left for the wards I approach the uncooperative consultant with two of my other senior colleagues. He persists in making excuses for his unhelpful behaviour, stressing that he is hard enough worked as it is without taking over these additional patients. We too are over-worked. This is not going to end well: 'Look,' I tell him, pointing my finger (never point, never point, NEVER POINT) at his chest, angry now as the painful belt of shingles tightens around *my* chest. I add: 'If you don't get a grip and sort yourself out I'm going to report this to the medical director.'

My voice is tense. To him my accent sounds like someone about to pull out a broadsword. He's looking at me as if my face is painted in woad. In my head it's as if I'm lamely saying: *I'll get my big brother onto you.* I shouldn't have bothered threatening to call the medical director. I should have gone straight to the phone.

Later that night the director phones me. He says I should not have argued with this colleague and that I should apologise to him. He says this too: 'Don't be surprised if he reports you to the GMC: he's very litigious.'

Not another one! And so I spend another month seeing some-times forty patients a day with those scorching marks on my chest healing, all the while waiting for a summons from the GMC.

He doesn't contact them. My apology is enough. Another apology. But his unhelpful attitude is never really challenged. Nothing is done about it. Not that I'm made aware of. He has not been held to account. That I'm not surprised is the saddest part of this story. The NHS is crumbling. Then back at the clinic another joker comes in: 'You're no relation to Dr Quinn, medicine woman?'

I'm dictating a letter. I generally do this in front of a patient immediately after we have concluded our discussion. That way the patient can correct you if there are any obvious errors of fact. You are recapitulating what has been said and I think the patients like this. They are also aware that there is no hidden agenda: they are hearing what you are thinking and have the additional reassurance that you will send them a copy.

I'm very aware as I dictate that I'm talking to one of our secretaries, who will transcribe the tape. Some of my colleagues have their dictation send abroad (to India, I think) to be transcribed. They get the letters back for signing and many complain of mistakes such as 'the patient was terminally ill and Cheyne-Stoking' turned into 'the patient was terminally ill and chain smoking', that kind of thing. (Cheyne-Stokes respirations are alternate fast breathing followed by no breathing and are often the harbinger of imminent death. Folks with the Cheyne-Stokes are not on the smokes.)

Maybe my letters are not sent abroad because I'm Glaswegian: even the locals affect a struggle to understand what I'm saying. I fight with those automated answering machines that ask: 'Did you want switchboard?'

'Yes, yes, switchboard, I want switchboard.'

'Connecting you to the mortuary.'

This is why I've been allowed to retain the services of our secretariat. I'm aware they have to sit and listen to my stuff and make sense of it: 'How are you spelling phaeochromocytoma, Dr Quin?'

When a parent comes in to see me accompanied by a young child, I'm always impressed by the inevitable fascination the dictating machine has for the kid. To cheer up my secretaries I'll often ask the child to say 'hello' to them on tape. Some of the youngsters love doing this and are duly amazed to hear their voices on playback. Others turn away shyly.

Sometimes I'll change my accent, do impersonations just to keep the secretaries amused. I think I heard Martin Amis on the radio one time mentioning people with 'thick' regional accents. I assume he meant 'pronounced'. Some use the word 'strong' when they describe another's accent, in the same disdainful way one might describe a mephitic blue cheese as 'strong'. Martin, of course, has a pronounced, indeed a strong, Oxbridge accent. A *thick* accent, some might say. So I'll sometimes do a Martin when dictating: 'Ah, a lettah to the GP. I reviewed this men at my clinic today. Ahm show he is suffing from ihr-ectile dysfunction and this, ah, I think mehtters deeply to him. Ken you prescribe him some Vay-agrah.'

Or I might drop into some Cockney or Farage estuary. Sometimes I'm pushing on so fast in order to see all the patients waiting I find myself sneezing inadvertently onto the tape and try as I might to delete this I find that I'm too squeezed for time and so apologise profusely to the hidden secretary. Rarely, after a particularly difficult conversation, I will start the letter off seriously and then subvert it, a first draft never to be sent out, an explosion of angst to be shared only between the secretary and myself:

Dear GP,

I reviewed this ungrateful bastard at the clinic again today. As usual he regaled me with a long list of imaginary symptoms, none of which have an organic basis. His manner was sullen. He swore at me with great regularity. I told him, as ever, to fuck the fuck off out of it. I'm grateful for you continuing his care.

My longest-serving secretary was Viv, a triplet; she got my gags. Viv answered all the patient calls with great politeness and sensitivity. I had virtually no need to correct any of her letters over many years. And then she developed cancer. My wife and I saw her at the hospice as she was dying. She was in her late forties.

I recall my wife and I walking home together in shock after we saw her for the last time and holding onto each other as if we might fall. A few months later I took her grieving husband on a trip out to Berlin. He could barely walk 500 yards. The blow was physical.

Sometimes the other secretaries make me listen in to a colleague's dictation. They're having a problem understanding what is being said. They switch the tape on and I listen in: '*Ayesawthismanwithhistiocytosisexandheisfeelinggrooostig.*'

The secretaries stare at me in incomprehension and ask: 'What's he saying?'

I give it a try: 'I think he is saying... "I saw this man"... uhm... with "histiocytosis X" and... ah... "he is feeling"... I'm not sure. Maybe "*Groostig*"?'

'Is that German?'

I enjoy having a bit of a carry-on with the secretaries when I go up to see them. I sign my letters and banter. They usually listen to the radio as they type and when Elton comes on I'll point out the inconsistencies of him going out for a fight on a Saturday night: 'Elton John's old lady not giving a fig that he's out all night picking fights? She don't care? Nah, c'mon: that's just not right.'

They indulge me with cake and make the day that bit more tolerable. One of the many phones goes off: 'It's Paul again asking to speak with you, John.'

Paul has Klinefelter syndrome. He has an extra X chromosome. His cells have three sex chromosomes: he is XXY. The condition is commoner than we previously presumed and there are many undiagnosed men out there. Some patients have behavioural problems: it is said that there are not a few people with Klinefelter's in prison. They often have low testosterone levels and so there is an argument to top them up with injections to prevent osteoporosis. Low testosterone can cause thin bones. But the injections can exacerbate any anger issues. Paul has anger issues: 'Listen, you cunt. It's my neck again. It hurts like buggery. What are you gonna do about it?'

For the umpteenth time I express sympathy and explain that I'm his endocrinologist and that he sees the rheumatologists for his neck problem: 'Yeah, fobbing me off again. That's all you doctors do. Fob us off. Fuck me... I'm poggered.'

Poggered?

'Yeah, mate, poggered. And cunts like you can do nothing about it.'

Maybe that's medicine in a nutshell. Cunts like us can do nothing for the poggered. I wind up with: 'Well, I'm sorry Paul. It's always nice to speak with you.'

All the while the secretaries are listening in and watching me gurn down the phone unseeingly to Paul. Some futurologists, some optimists, are keen on us consulting by Skype. I'm not a fan of the idea of Skyping patients like Paul. Life is too short to Skype the likes of Paul. I look up 'poggered' on Google. It says: 'A Romany Gypsy term meaning broken, ruined, damaged. A corruption of the Jewish/Russian word pogrom meaning devastated.'

That's what we should call the story of the NHS in the early twenty-first century: *Poggered.*

I meet another lad with Klinefelter's who is much nicer than Paul. He sits down and opens his shirt. 'I want to show you something!'

He's tattooed his chest wall. In large blue letters on his pectorals I can now read XXY.

'I did it just in case the hospital couldn't find my notes. I read that they can often go missing. Well, they can't miss that.' Pointing to those large initials above his nipples: XXY.

The Deanery continues to intrigue. One of the senior players, a pathologist, invites us to his gentlemen's club off Pall Mall: the Athenaeum. I've heard of it before, probably when I read Evelyn Waugh. The pathologist is pear-shaped, clipped in manner, catty but amusing. He, like some modern-day Samuel Johnson, regards me with gentle condescension, suspicious of Scotland and the Scots. He secretly worries that we harbour notions of independence and Republicanism, as with the Irish. He's right to be wary, of course. He seems rigorously certain that his Tory beliefs are flawless.

I head to Pall Mall. The building is in the neoclassical style and has an impressive Doric portico. The pathologist greets us in the upstairs library. We sit near the open fire and admire the dusty tomes no one ever reads. The portraits that line the walls strike one as having a startling indifference to technique or basic aesthetics. A waiter serves us drinks and the Dean blows another Louis Armstrong blast into his handkerchief and then picks up his glass of malt. I have a lowly beer, trying my best to appear unintimidated. This is made easier by the presence elsewhere of several wan members of the clergy. They sit with their arms folded gently across their laps and meekly sip at tea. They recall sitcom characters, people from the BBC world of the 1970s: the naff British TV of Dick Emery and *It Ain't Half Hot Mum*, when pop monsters like Jimmy Savile felt emboldened to go about their toxic business unchecked.

The food is forgettable. The pathologist tells us something of the history of the club. Founded in 1824. Dickens and Darwin were members. Ladies were allowed membership only as late as 2002. Later I read that Robert Louis Stevenson was a member and (help!) Jimmy Savile too: heroes and villains. Dinner over and the Dean gets his hanky out again: the evening ends with a mighty cheek-expanding Dizzy Gilles- pie of an explosion. I suspect he's about as comfortable here as I am.

I'm back at the clinic. The outpatient nurses are in a flap and barge into my office: 'Quick, we need help!'

I go outside with them and find a woman tearing around and talking in riddles. I manage to calm her and get her seated in my room. She is quite florid in complexion and her face is moon- shaped. She finds it hard to get out of a chair and I know this is because she has muscle wasting. She has a hump on the back of her neck. What we call a buffalo hump: another example of medicine's insensitivity with words. And she is obese. The older, wiser, but no more sensitive doctors of the past said that such patients looked like a lemon with four matchsticks stuck in it. I do not tell her this. She has Cushing's syndrome.

Cushing's was named after Harvey Cushing (1869–1939), who was from Ohio and was one of the fathers of neurosurgery – indeed, the Big Daddy. His eponymous syndrome is one in which the body makes excess amounts of steroid hormone. This happens in some cases because the pituitary gland makes too much of a hormone called ACTH (adrenocorticotrophic hormone) which stimulates the adrenal gland. A pituitary tumour causes this variety of the syndrome called (confusingly) Cushing's disease. These tumours are invariably benign; however, they are to be found in tiger coun- try, deep in the centre of the brain. Excess steroid causes muscle wasting, central abdominal obesity, high blood pressure and osteo- porosis, a bad combo, hence the unsubtle comparison to a lemon stuck with matchsticks. The condition must be treated, as it can kill due to its deleterious effect on blood pressure. Excess steroids have a dramatic effect on mood. They can make you, like our woman in the clinic, seriously manic. I take quite some time explaining to her that she's not going mad and that it is hormones that are doing this to her and that we can sort it out.

If the cause is excess ACTH then the cure can be effected by a transsphenoidal hypophysectomy: removal of the pituitary gland via the nose. I'm filled with awe at the idea of Harvey Cushing doing this before CT or MRI scanning was available. Basically he would have put his probe up someone's nose and then begun to blindly dissect. Unsurprisingly he ran into problems, such as causing a leak of cerebrospinal fluid or damaging the normal pituitary, thus rendering the patient hypopituitary, an underactive pituitary that would require the patient to be on replacement hormones. Or maybe doing both…

The investigative protocols for Cushing's remain highly complex and labour intensive. They can involve cannulation of both femoral veins in the groin and then repeated venous sampling from the head, neck and chest. Prior labelling of the sampling bottles is a key precautionary measure and this can easily go wrong.

In this lady's case the lesion was in fact in her adrenal glands, another sub-type of Cushing's syndrome: one gland had developed a benign tumour. In due course this was removed by keyhole surgery and she was effectively cured. Her bone density thickened after many months. Her moon-face was soon eclipsed; she regained her looks. Her mania settled, though like many she had a subsequent period of depression. She was fantastically grateful when this re-solved itself and I always looked forward to seeing her as evidence, as reassurance, that sometimes we get it right.

This mania caused by excess steroids could be dramatic. One man I met was being treated for HIV and he was inadvertently given some steroids by another team of specialists: these interacted with his HIV therapy, a now well-known scenario but back then little recognised. They were about to try to get a sample of his cerebro-spinal fluid as part of the investigation into his change of mental state when he reached over the bedside and grabbed the spinal needle. Imagine a small knitting needle. This he raised high and then, *wham*, stuck it in his neck. Miraculously he missed his carotid vessels by millimetres. Now you know why some endocrinologists got a tad anxious when they heard that Trump was put on high-dose steroid *and* an antiviral for his Covid-19.

Later I heard about another woman cared for elsewhere who was rendered Cushingoid in a similar manner via an HIV drug interaction. She went to her lawyers and subsequently received a substantial settlement.

Steroids can be very tricky. People abuse them, of course; in Brighton they call them 'Muscle Marys'. Guys who use anabolic steroids to buff up their six-packs. One problem: your nuts shrink. Surprisingly there were not a few who seemed to accept this trade-off.

I'm asked to be an independent opinion by a coroner on a case elsewhere in the country. A nineteen-year-old girl has died. The family of the girl is very keen to know that the lessons of her death be publicised. They are not seeking compensation; they do not wish for those who cared for her to be prosecuted. This is an important point to note as of late doctors and healthcare workers have been prosecuted for manslaughter, most recently an optometrist given a two-year suspended prison sentence for missing the rare diagnosis of a neuroblastoma, later overturned on appeal. Many in medicine see this development, the sentencing of healthcare workers for mistakes, as highly worrying in an environment of cutbacks. Ophthalmoscopes (to take a quotidian example) are frequently not to be found in A+E departments. They've been stolen. So it is highly likely that, in their absence, mistakes will be made, more diagnoses will be missed.

I look into the details of the girl's sad case. She had been unwell for some time and her doctor thought the diagnosis was an eating disorder, that she had anorexia nervosa. The doctor concluded this was the cause of the girl's extensive weight loss. Two blood samples sent by the doctor revealed low sodium levels: the girl was low in salt. The family stated categorically that she craved salt and drank directly from a bottle of dark soy sauce at breakfast time. And she herself was getting darker: her skin was changing in hue, as if she were being tanned without being in the sun. They had not been on holiday. All this information – the low serum sodium, the craving for salt, the weight loss, the skin pigmentation – all these features suggested a diagnosis of Addison's disease.

Addison's is a life-threatening deficiency of cortisol production. Just as patients with Cushing's syndrome make too much cortisol, so Addisonian patients make too little. Tragically the condition is easily missed and can be fatal. Famously JFK had Addison's and had to wait until he was nearly at death's door before it was diagnosed, coincidentally when he was in Britain. The girl eventually collapsed and was brought to A+E, where she could not be resuscitated. This was truly awful. I agreed with the senior endocrinologist review-ing her case: the most likely diagnosis was Addison's. If it had been diagnosed, she would have been started on steroids and she would have lived.

A national warning was duly sent out to all GPs asking that they be aware of the condition given the ease of missing the signs and the terrible consequences. That dreadful detail about soy sauce for breakfast stays with me. Perhaps unsurprisingly I'm frightened of missing the diagnosis. This paranoia in time becomes a not-insignificant burden.

A Friday afternoon and, ward work completed, handover for the weekend performed, I'm getting ready to go home and welcome Danvers, now forgiving of the Kylie Minogue wind-up and the Stuart Sutcliffe painting debacle. He and his wife have flown 500 miles down to see us from Glasgow. We are due to meet at five in the evening, close of play. At 3 p.m. I get an email from our biochemistry department saying they have received a sample that morning from a young man of about eighteen called Luke who would appear to have Addison's. His morning cortisol is below twenty. This is highly alarming. This is not what I want to hear on a Friday afternoon.

My throat dries when I'm told the result. A morning cortisol should be at least over 200. Most people, first thing, can get it over 500. I speak to the nurse who took blood from Luke. Her suspicions have made the diagnosis. Nurses, and midwives, often make diagnoses: the public needs to know this, needs to reward them appropriately. She says the boy has been losing weight and cutting back on his usual insulin dosage.

He's got diabetes too. People with Type 1 diabetes are more at risk of Addison's because both are autoimmune conditions where the body makes antibodies to its own tissue. We have very little idea why the body does this, but we do know it can be fatal. I remember poor Richard's voice, Richard after his dive over the cliffs, thinking to himself in his tent: *I'm destroying myself, ah well.* I look up the boy's phone number on the computer (great, it's there) and call him. Then there's the doot-doot-doot of the unavailable tone.

Help. It's now quarter past three. I try his GP and wait another fifteen minutes before being told that that's the only contact number they have for him. Daily I'm struck by how many people do not leave any kind of current contact number for their GP to use. Then I have a brainwave. I'll write out a prescription for some steroid, catch a cab to his address and hand the script to either Luke or his mum. I'll be back well in time for Danvers and his wife.

Luke's house is just outside the city, but not too far. I check my pockets; just enough cash to pay the taxi driver there and back. Who then does his best to get us there as quickly as possible. I jump out the cab once we get to Luke's street and I run up to the door and ring the bell. A dark shape appears at the frosted glass. Great, somebody's at home. A woman opens the door narrowly and I rapidly ask her: 'Are you Luke's mother?'

'Who?'

'Luke Pollock. He lives here, doesn't he? I'm his doctor at the hospital and it's an emergency: he needs this drug now.'

I'm showing her a tatty green piece of paper that has my writing asking the pharmacist to prescribe life-saving hydrocortisone, fifteen milligrams to be taken in the morning and ten for the evening.

'No, I'm really sorry, there's no one of that name who lives here. I'm really sorry to upset you. Is it that bad?'

Yes, it is that bad: it's very bad. Now it is four o'clock on a Friday afternoon and I've got a life-threatening situation with no lead as to how I can get a hold of this young guy and I've got visitors who will have to sit around for an age waiting for me. Shit. I contemplate phoning the police. Maybe they can trace him. Didn't he work for a supermarket somewhere in London? Asda, was it? How many Asdas are there in London? Jesus. That whittles down the chances of finding him from, oh, one in 10 million to one in 1 million maybe.

I'm back in my office and beginning to despair when it dawns on me to try the GP again, maybe he's got Luke's mum's number.

I remember now that his mum is due to remarry. Soon. She mentioned taking Luke to the honeymoon. Where was it again? I rack my memory... uhm, yes... got it! Australia! But say he has gone already? Oh, hell. Do I need to call the Australian embassy? I've had enough of Australian officialdom for one lifetime. Do we need the ambassador to get involved? It's now four-thirty in the afternoon and I'm near panic. The GP has her number! I call her and she answers, she's in, it's her: 'Is this really that important? I'm at work.'

'I'm afraid it is. Where is Luke just now?'

'He's at a theme park in the Midlands. But he's back tomorrow: should I call him?'

'Yes, please. Please! And tell him to get a friend to drive him home. Can he come up to see me tomorrow or can you pop up just now to get the prescription?'

'I can pop up. Is it *really* that serious? I'm flying to Brisbane next week to get married.'

'I'll tell you more when you get up here.'

She arrives just before five and I have time to call Danvers to say that I'll be half an hour late. The Friday panic phenomenon is so regular in medicine as to be a cliché of the profession. Mum arrives and she is wearing a pair of Dr Martens boots. Not for the last time I'm struck by her laid-back manner. I give her the prescription. She is incredulous that I went up to their house by cab. I say: 'But it isn't your house, is it? Maybe a mistake when Luke was registering with us?'

'Oh, no, it is our house.'

She is a polite, confident lady, looking forward to happiness at the altar. She explains: 'Yes, that *is* our house. It's up for rent. I'm going to sell it and maybe move out to Oz. That lady you met was the person renting it.'

'She couldn't have recognised your surname then?'

'I guess probably not. But look… is this *really* life-threatening, this thing that Luke has?'

I nod. I'm thinking of that nineteen-year-old girl, the empty bottles of soy sauce on the breakfast table, the failed resuscitation. She takes the prescription and calls Luke in front of me. He has a new mobile phone but like most young people doesn't think to update us with this information because, well, because he's young, and the young (rightly) don't think too much about death. He is a kid and his head is full of theme parks. This is as it should be if you're young. Luke is en route up north, but he will turn back.

I make it home before six and meet my friends. Danvers cheers me up by telling me his outrageous story about the nurse who thinks he can communicate with the deaf by imitating their vocalisations. I'm crying with laughter as he does his impersonation. We eat well at a restaurant not far from our house and after finishing dinner Danvers gets up to go to the bathroom. Where he finds a girl who was at the table next to us. Finds her spark out on the floor, blood oozing from her occiput. He yells for help.

Fuck. Will this mad day ever end?

We get her in an ambulance. Maybe she's fainted, but maybe she's had a fit; she needs to be assessed up at the hospital. We stagger home. The next day I call A+E. She'd only fainted. Life will go on for her.

16

THE ABSOLUT VODKA ART PRIZE

Life goes on for me too, and I want to write. My first proper assign-
ment was back in 1999: that review of Stacy Schiff's biography of
Vera Nabokov in *The Guardian*. I heard the news of its acceptance
when I was walking around a fast-gentrifying Prenzlauer Berg in
Berlin. I punched the Berliner Luft as I bounced down Schönhauser
Allee. Published in a national newspaper! I called my parents and
they bought a copy. Cut the article out. Hung it in the lavatory.
You're no Mozart.

We had hired an apartment there in Prenzlauer Berg for a couple
of weeks and walked the undivided city, had food in bright new
Thai restaurants, beers in Russian-themed cafés with names like
Gagarin and Pasternak. We sat outside in the sun across from a
cylindrical water tower where the Nazis once tortured communists
in a basement; this had now been converted into a block of flats.
The city was full of trees. Pink cherry blossoms lined Lottumstrasse.
The city's cultural life was also blooming. The end of the twentieth
century saw a boom in the electronic music scene; visual artists
were beginning to leave London too for Berlin with its outsized,
and much cheaper, studios.

The walls in this part of Berlin still bore bullet-hole scars; even the museums had chunks gouged out of their Greek columns courtesy of the Red Army. A friend, the French conceptual painter Pierre Millotte, was looking after our own place back in Brighton. Later Pierre sends us two canvases to commemorate our holidays. I was thirty-eight years old that year and I wanted to write about art.

I started to pitch to magazines suggesting reviews, and *The Lancet* and the *British Medical Journal* accept some more articles on art and literature. I'm happy with these, particularly when I slip some mildly subversive references to popular culture past the editors, but I crave publication in non-medical journals, the usual fantasies of being published in the likes of *Artforum* or the *New Yorker*. Having imaginary chats with the fact checkers at the *New Yorker*: does the earth rotate from east to west or west to east? What is the correct spelling of amitriptyline? Three 'i's. But I don't want to be writing about amitriptyline, I want to be writing about paintings.

Proper art reviewing begins with acceptance of work by the Scottish arts publication *MAP*. Shortly after that I get an article in an internationally sold magazine called *contemporary*: note the modernist use of the lower case, a then in-vogue appropriation of e e cummings's style. The thrill of seeing a piece in print, on the racks of a newsagent, becomes addictive. I try for a glossy and hit pay dirt when the highly attractive *Zembla*, a new magazine dedicated to contemporary fiction, accepts a proposal to run an interview with the publisher John Calder.

Calder had been a hero of mine for years. My dad, as a young man then in his twenties, bought many books published by Calder. This would have been in the early 1960s. His select library was my first exposure to Beckett. Dad got his hands on many of the banned books from those times, now classics: Hubert Selby Jr's *Last Exit to Brooklyn*, the novels of Alex Trocchi, Burroughs, all via John Calder. That Calder was a fellow Scot added my fascination. I was impressed that he was still alive, still publishing, even well into his seventies. His offices were on The Cut, near Waterloo Station, close to a green-tiled fish restaurant that I'd been in before.

He was wearing a dark pinstriped three-piece suit, the waistcoat straining somewhat, black shoes and sky-blue socks. We descended a stairwell to his office, where we drank coffee and chatted. In manner he had something of the Edinburgh advocate about him: assured, combative if necessary – perhaps no surprise given his own dealings with the legal profession, his challenges against censorship, his successes against those who would restrict free speech. We talked for over an hour. The conversation ranged widely: there was his attempt to create a Scottish Glyndebourne at Ledlanet; his laconic meetings with Sam the Man; his tolerance of Alex the Junkie and the battle between Trocchi and Hugh MacDiarmid at the Edinburgh Festival in the early '60s, the one where Hugh called Alex 'cosmopolitan scum'. We talked too about his championing of Ann Quin and her sad death in Brighton. Calder was nearing eighty and despite his manifest unfitness was still robust in mind. He had known wild times.

I wrote up the interview, submitted the piece to *Zembla* and was chuffed as a preening peacock to hear that it would be out in the next edition. It looked great stacked at the newsagent's. The magazine was expensively printed with glossy pages and had a beautiful actress on the cover. I skimmed through the issue looking for my work. Someone had told me that British Airways were giving out complimentary copies of *Zembla* to business-class passengers. Ah, here it was! Great: a double spread. Text looks fine, photographs, lovely. But wait, what's this? *John Calder by David Franks*. David who? David... *oh fuck, naw!*

No. No, no, no. They've published my piece with the wrong author's name! My mind imploding: no one will ever know it was *me* who wrote this! Welcome to the world of the freelancer, Dr Quin. *Zembla* issued a small apology in the next issue and, as it sold poorly, ceased publication the next year.

The movement of the arts from London to Berlin continues apace during the early 2000s. I spend more time out there and start writing for *ArtReview*. Chris Ofili commissions a piece for one of his gorgeous monographs. The book is a silver and cobalt-blue affair: my writing references religion and the Old Firm.

We're invited to a small party in Hanover to celebrate his show. In a corner Chris is wearing headphones, fiddling with a set of decks. Jonathan Meese and Peter Doig and Tal R and Daniel Richter and Isaac Julien are here; the crowd is jiving to a (then) groovy tune by Franz Ferdinand. That one about the Transmission party, the one where 'we're with our friends, they're oh so arty'. Oh, yeah. And then, as the music stops, as I take the last sips of a cocktail, I realise, I remember, that I'm on call for admissions in A+E next weekend and will be working twelve days straight. I decide on another beer.

Back in Berlin, still on annual leave, I get a call from the hospital managers as I walk down Friedrichstrasse: 'Hi John, just wondering if you can help out with the bed-state?'

Brighton calling: there are problems with capacity. We do not have enough beds for our patients. Many elderly inpatients can't be discharged because their homes are not fit for purpose: they need railings, lifts and so on. They are labelled, cruelly, as 'bed-blockers'. We meet them on our rounds and say a gentle hello. They need no medical input. We meet them more regularly than our own parents, our own partners. Our managers now insist on *daily* consultant-led ward rounds. In time they even ask for two a day. A ward round generally takes up about three to four hours. *Fit them in between clinics.*

No money is forthcoming to help the situation: the money is being spent on something else. We have trouble getting locums, posts are unfilled and clinics cancelled. The government's desire to see the NHS survive is in serious question. Brickbats are thrown at the service by the press. Complaints are increasing at a frightening rate. Those on the front line spend more and more time apologising, placating. Reports come in of scandals at other hospitals. This can't go on much longer.

I'm back in west Berlin in 2010. A bottle of white wine, a table made of wood, as Iggy Pop would have it. We're having dinner at the Paris Bar courtesy of the gallery Contemporary Fine Arts, a celebration for the American artist Julian Schnabel. I'm not a fan but maybe there is such a thing as a free meal after all, at least in the art world. We eat fatty steak and chips and drink rough Grenache after the white. Sarah Lucas, Martin Kippenberger and the aforementioned Daniel Richter cover the walls in works, salon-style. And there are photographs by Damien Hirst and Dash Snow, there's a Meese scrawl, a Doig. The Doig is a swiftly executed watercolour of Truman Capote wearing a black hat and a red cape. A plastic V2 rocket is suspended from the ceiling, as is a tatty light box by Angus Fairhurst that reads: *Stand Still and Rot.* My mind wanders from the glamour of the event after reading this portent and it strikes me that this is what our government seems to be telling the NHS. Stand still and rot.

We talk to the gallery owner, Nicole. Her husband Bruno is getting merrily pished with Schnabel over in a corner; she doesn't want him to start singing. Bruno loves performing in public: usually something from Iggy's *The Idiot*. I'm hoping he will. Then my mood flattens when I remember that I've got to fly back and do five clinics and five ward rounds in five days next week. With no registrar – he's on paternity leave – no assistance.

The 'juniors' are restive. They struggle to pay off their student debts. We got grants in my day. We had no real excuse for debt other than beer. When I was a student my bank manager refused to allow me any more than £200 as an overdraft. After I graduated I wanted to go on a holiday before starting work. The bank refused to extend my overdraft unless I could produce some exam prize money I'd won. Can't it wait until they mail it to me? *No, no, go get it from them.* The Clydesdale Bank made me, right there and then, head up to an office at the university. I had to ask them: please, can you give me my prize money? Eh, now please, if you can. I closed my account after my first pay cheque.

Nowadays newly qualified doctors are up to £70,000 in debt. They hate the new shift systems. The hours overall are better but the work is more intense because modern medicine is more effective than the 1980s, the interventions more successful. Sickness rates are on the rise. Being told you have no registrar for the round today comes as no surprise. Many consultants end up doing ward rounds alone. No trainees, no nurses: just you and a trolley full of case notes.

Revising the paragraph above for the first time I took a break and glanced at my Twitter feed. Margaret McCartney had replaced Liam Farrell at the *BMJ*. Her tweets, her articles were becoming ever more trenchant. I retweeted her comment from 10 September 2016. She said, simply, this: *I think the NHS is being wilfully destroyed.*

I'm in Stockholm, 2011, for the Absolut Vodka Art Prize ceremony.

I've interviewed the winner, the very talented Albanian artist Anri Sala, and I'm now wearing my long unwanted, long under-used tuxedo. No obvious moth bites. We're sipping on tart citric cocktails fuelled by Absolut and sitting at a table with the great and the good. My neighbours are, to my right, Mr Ricard (the pastis company's man in Europe) and, to my left, a startlingly impressive couple, a pair of Swedish diplomats. What the hell am I doing here?

Dinner over and the ceremony begins. The bigwigs congratulate Anri: the music strikes up, Franz Ferdinand again; they really *are* so arty. Anri grabs me and introduces me to his sister.

We get chatting and are quick to ask each other what we do and where we are working. Turns out she is a nuclear medicine consultant based in Oxford. We laugh at the improbability of two doctors being at the Absolut Art Prize.

Back the following week at clinic and I'm trying to be gently insistent to yet another young man who has a normal testosterone level that he does not need testosterone. He thinks his tackle isn't impressive enough. Like a couple of other young men I've been asked to see at the clinic, he thinks his cock should be bigger. His cock is quite normal on examination. He's probably watching too much pornography. These guys unfairly compare themselves with the priapic male stars. I do not vocalise this suspicion, but it is clear I can't help him. Like the others, he storms out after half an hour. Half an hour when I could have been reassuring that young mother with thyroid cancer sitting patiently outside.

There's a pattern emerging here. I'm in Istanbul in late 2012 at a rooftop bar after midnight with a heart-stopping view over the

Golden Horn. I'm sipping milk-coloured raki with a new friend, Rüdiger, a Berliner who works at *Der Tagesspiegel*. We have spent the day with one of the Koç family, Mehmet, the younger son, who deals with the art side of the business. He has opened a new gallery on İstiklal Caddesi. His place across the Bosporus is like something from a Bond movie. Rüdiger and I compare notes about Mehmet's collection, exquisite pieces that line his walls. The bathroom is hilarious, what with its explicit photographic works. Back in the dining room I rejoin the group and ask Rüdiger: is that a real Grosz? Jings: it is! And those wild works that decorate the loo: how is that possible in an Islamic country? Could he get into trouble with this guy Erdoğan?

And then I'm back home again in A+E for the run-up to Christmas. The emergency department is busy. A TV soap opera story about overdoses has led to some copycat admissions. And the secretaries have received a complaint. *You didn't tell me that this side effect might happen.* Yes, I did. Look, here's a copy of the letter I sent you to prove it.

In my fifties I spend way too much of the precious time I have left on earth with sociopaths or psychopaths or whatever you want to call them. The personality disordered, that 1 per cent or so of humanity. What at any other time in history people would call 'wankers'. Wankers have become empowered by the complaints procedures, the disciplinary processes and the more feral aspects of the media. But we have to take their baseless whining seriously; we have to be polite to them. The days when they could be safely escorted off the premises have long gone.

The personality disordered bleat 'I'll be in touch with my MP' or 'You'll be hearing from my solicitor/the *Daily Mail/The One Show*'.

Wankers make up less than one in a hundred people we see, but they are time-consuming, wearying and wearing.

Smiling benignly at someone who has just called you a cunt (because you don't think there are any rational grounds for prescribing him some enormously expensive medication) gets tougher and tougher as the years pile on: your face pleads for understanding, you bear a rigidly fixed rictus, as if your cheeks had been zapped hourly with shots of Botox. But here's the sad truth: these assholes are memorable.

Ninety-nine per cent of people we see are lovely: they are people like you and me. Some are even kind enough to leave you chocolates, a book, a CD, a bottle of Châteauneuf-du-Pape, that aforementioned Old Pulteney after you've finished their care. But here's a sad fact: not infrequently these kind folks don't fix themselves in memory *precisely* because they are so nice, so unprepossessing. They are modest; they say thoughtfully: *You're a busy man, Doctor.*

It's the aggressive ones who stick in the mind; they're the tossers you have nightmares about, the ones you want to go all Travis Bickle on: *Are you talking to me?*

And here's the deal about psychopaths: you can't say this to them: 'Do you know that you are a psychopath?' You can't diagnose them as such. You can't label them. You can't say to someone who is calling you a cunt: 'Cut that out, you, you... *psychopath*.' Hell mend you if you actually label someone a psychopath.

A psycho would complain if you called them a psycho. That would set in motion a chain of events causing serious grief: you would probably be disciplined by your hospital management for being 'rude'; you might be reported to the GMC; you might get stabbed as well. I've never heard of a doctor telling a patient straight out: *You're psychopathic. Mate... you're a psycho.*

Physicians are faced with a lot more psychiatric patients these days given the reduction in psychiatric bed numbers. Mad people turn up at A+E raving and cursing because of failed care-in-the-community programmes. Whose fault is that? Money-saving, austerity-package, advanced-consumer-choice, couldn't-give-a-fuck hyper-capitalism.

The Powers That Be are worried about recruitment into A+E. They don't know how we might attract doctors and nurses to come and work with empowered psychopaths who want to stab you.

Here's two more individuals you might describe as 'challenging'.

CASE ONE

When I was an SHO back in the 1980s there was a guy in his thirties who would turn up to A+E around midnight dressed in a tuxedo. He would tell you some cock-and-bull story about vomiting up blood. Now if you ever, for some bizarre reason, crave admission to hospital all you need to do is tell the admissions team you've vomited up blood, you've had a *haematemesis*. But don't use that word because the docs will immediately become suspicious. Just say: 'I've vomited up some blood' and you'll be in a bed with a line in your arm before you know it. Quite why you would *want* to be admitted to a hospital if you are well remains one of life's great mysteries. Some can be explained: an unloved teenager struggling with diabetes, her mum in jail and dad off whoring it in Thailand, she might just prefer the love and attention in hospital; ditto a vagrant craving some heat in the winter. But what about this guy in the tuxedo? What kind of weirdo is he? He gets admitted.

And then, once safely tucked in a bed, he presses the call button for a nurse and when she arrives he thumps her. Punches her square in the face. That's right. Punches a young woman in the face. Eventually a photograph of *his* face would be in every A+E in the UK. One hopes he no longer exists. Psychiatrists have trouble with the word *evil*. You'll never read this in someone's case notes – Diagnosis: Evil. That guy was evil. Maybe, rarely, we should write this at the end of a clerk-in: Impression: Evil.

CASE TWO

A man with HIV: the virus is under control. His life expectancy on his protease inhibitors may be even longer than average. But he is also taking a mixed bag of hormones: testosterone, hydrocortisone, thyroxine and growth hormone. I'm immediately sceptical. With my polite poker face now on I ask: 'Can you tell me why you're on these?'

'You can ask but I'm not going to tell you.'

'Uh huh. OK. Can I ask who started you on these drugs?'

'You can ask but I'm not going to tell you.'

'It might help me to understand your case better...'

'Fine. All right, if you insist. It was a consultant in another city.'

'Can I ask who it was?'

'You can ask but again I'm not going to tell you.'

'OK. Uhm... can I ask you why not?'

'Because then you will write to them and I don't want you to do that.'

'But it would help me to find out what their rationale was in starting these treatments.'

'No! You would just want to stop them and you'd say they were too expensive. I know your type.'

He knows my 'type'. I spend at least ten minutes patiently explaining that cost is *not* the key issue here and that these drugs, these hormones, can do significant harm if they are not indicated, but it's useless. He slams his newspaper on my desk and storms out. Most of my colleagues come across a very similar type of scenario, the angry exit, the impatient patient, the unreasonable demand, at least once a month.

Support from colleagues is essential. I'm lucky to have many who are a model of professionalism. They are what you would want were you to fall ill and need their care. I'm with Nicky in London. She is one of the best doctors I know: unflappable, focused, patient, highly organised, a motivator; she's a true leader. We have finished a Deanery meeting and have enough time to visit a tony art gallery before it closes at six.

We walk up a set of rickety old wooden steps and see thirteen spectacular paintings by Chris Ofili, his riff on the apostles and a little-known early drawing by Andy Warhol. Nicky is hugely impressed. I mention that I've got something in this month's *ArtReview* and she shocks me by saying that it was her grandfather, Richard, a doctor himself, who set up the magazine back in 1949. The first edition was designed by his wife, Nicky's grandmother, Eileen Mayo. Richard did all this after he retired. He was a GP. I'm inspired to hear this. We get talking about doctors and the arts and writing. I tell her the story of Patrick Ireland. Patrick is a hero of mine. Patrick was a doctor too and he's a *real* art writer.

Patrick Ireland is not his real name. I like fake names: Jock Scot, Maxwell Park, Fay Fife. Patrick's *real* name is Brian O'Doherty and he was born in 1928. He grew up in Dublin and studied medicine there, worked at Harvard doing medical research and then (abracadabra) auditioned for a job as a TV presenter and found himself doing interviews with Chagall, Walter Gropius, Stuart Davis. Years ago, before we could afford taking a punt on a print or a painting, my wife and I bought a large poster of *Swing Landscape* by Stuart Davis and got it framed, pomo '80s style, in aluminium. The thing dominated the tiny living room in our first flat. This is O'Doherty describing Davis in a bumper book of his writings: 'He looked like someone who was going to go and shoot craps any minute.'

O'Doherty's essays inspire. In so many words he's telling me that I need to up my game as a writer about art. He says that Stuart Davis had

a classic spirit, a spirit of the sort that could find some principle of eternal order in the neon wilderness of Times Square. He searched disorder for its underlying principle. Not long before his death, he told me: 'The value of impermanence is to call attention to the permanent.' It becomes his epitaph.

Searching disorder for its underlying principle: that statement could equally as well apply to life in A+E, in acute medicine. Soon after reading this I'm childishly chuffed to get an article on Roland Barthes accepted by *ArtReview*. I learn that O'Doherty commissioned Barthes to write his famous 'Death of the Author' essay for *Aspen* magazine back in 1967. O'Doherty then went on to write his seminal take on the new style of art gallery: *Inside the White Cube*.

Upset at the events of Bloody Sunday in 1972, O'Doherty began to sign his own artworks as 'Patrick Ireland'. He makes an ECG portrait of Marcel Duchamp and then gets shortlisted for the Booker Prize in 1992. In 2008 he kills off Patrick Ireland in recognition of the Northern Ireland peace process. O'Doherty is the epitome of doctor as critic, as artist; he chased both rabbits. Patrick Ireland may be dead but Brian O'Doherty, now in his nineties, is still alive and well in America.

Chris, one of the older cardiologists, is coming up for retirement. In O'Doherty's words he calls attention to the permanent by giving me his copy of Bulgakov's *A Young Doctor's Notebook* and says: 'This will bring it all back to you.'

He's right, it does. I'm struck by the weather in Bulgakov's stories: it's always a blizzard outside as he rides to the rescue of some poor woman trapped in labour with a transverse lie. The winds howl and a whiteout beckons him to oblivion.

And as Chris said, the memories of being a naïve young doctor flood back: not so many blizzards, for sure, but those mad nights getting out of bed after being shocked awake by the EEEE-EEEE-EEEE and putting my clothes back on again, the clammy feeling of pulling the previous day's pair of socks on, the stickiness around the collar of yesterday's shirt, the decision not to bother with a tie because, well, who cares at three in the morning? And then the walk outside in the darkness between the wards with the rain pouring down on you, lashing so it is.

You are a merry wanderer of the night, and now you're soaking wet and the wind whips up and cuffs you on the face. Some imp of the perverse from on high has poured down a full bucket of water on top of your head.

Thankfully the call is not to some labouring Russian mama but to a man dying from chronic obstructive airways disease and you know that, yes, he's had his time, he's in his late seventies and the many packs of Rothman's or whatever have done for him. You reach the ward and get a syringe and needle out in order to pierce his radial artery and do a blood gas estimation. The machine is in a small cupboard-like space with walls splattered with the spent blood of others. It's a room recalling images of a quite different red and white world, another dimly degraded garage-like place, seen in those crazed images of the St Valentine's Day Massacre and its aftermath. The man's oxygen level is critical, his carbon dioxide level sky-high because he's not blowing it off. He's a *blue bloater*. There's no way you can transfer him elsewhere for ventilation: no one would have him.

And so you consult your formulary, just like Bulgakov does when faced with his cases of syphilis, and you look for something that will make this poor man breathe. And you come up with… nikethamide. But wait, doesn't nikethamide make people fit? Let's not use that. Then you remember doxapram, yes, Dopram as it is marketed. Just the job. You hitch him up to an infusion and sneak out the ward and get soaked again by another deluge in the night. And finally you get out of that clinging shirt, those bogging socks, and sink, sink deep, deep, just like Bulgakov, into sleep. Boy, did Bulgakov love his sleep. Doctors the world over worship sleep: they value sleep. Doctors love a good kip. Forget all that Nabokovian nonsense about sleep meaning you are losing consciousness: Nabokov never knew about being called out to work in the wind and the rain and the snow, never knew walking in the cold early hours like Bulgakov, like, like… *me*! Nabokov, with his well-publicised insomnia, never knew how to love sleep. His loss.

But doxapram causes panic attacks and tremors and then around 4 a.m. you jerk awake after the EEEE-EEEE-EEEE of the bleep goes into overdrive. 'Your man is breathing now,' the nurse says, 'but he's jumping out of bed and wanting to go home and you'd better come back over to sort him out. Can we sedate him meantime?'

Sedation? That'll be a no. That will kill him. Sedation kills a blue bloater. First do no harm. So you head back out into the storm.

Mr Bulgakov has a propensity for ellipsis that's catching… maybe it's an infectious disease for writers… maybe Mr Céline, yet another doctor/writer, caught it from him too… I don't know, but it's a form that has always attracted me… maybe it's *the* form for doctor writers... say everything as fast as possible... you're running around all the time... every morning up at dawn with the tramps, the jakeys, the down-and-outs... bolting down food when you can get it... pissing quickly in between seeing patients even when you're worried about the remote possibility of a terminal dribble heading down your leg... Have I?... Has it stained my trousers?... Let's have a quick look down there... no, no, it's fine... onwards.

I like the fact that as a houseman Bulgakov would consult his textbooks and say: 'I'll be back in a minute, just need a cigarette.' Top move. I'd say something similar to a registrar on the phone: give me a second, I've got some toast on... and then you check on the internet after he's asked you if there's been any malaria in Papua New Guinea or Ebola in Senegal because, well, it's 3 a.m. and some-one has flown back from there with a fever and is now in A+E...

He likes exclamation marks too, does Mr Bulgakov! As with his early experiences doing version (turning babies in the womb), it was not the case of see one, do one, teach one, the much-criticised teaching mantra still under attack in the twenty-first century. No, no! For Mr Bulgakov, for me too, it was see none, do one, do anoth-er one, get used to it, son! Well, everything was grim back in 1917! Ditto medicine back in 1983! Medicine: it's always grim!

Bulgakov would try his best, mind and, guess what? He'd do fine, every time he'd come up smiling! The midwives would say stuff like: 'That was brilliant, Doctor!'

And yet in other moments, flushed with anger, Bulgakov would say crazy things like: 'Shut up, woman!' He'd say this to a ghastly interfering relative. They got away with so much, those old doctors. Years later and I'm in a Berlin cinema watching King Vidor's 1938 movie of A. J. Cronin's *The Citadel*. At one point the doctor hero slaps a woman in the face. He diagnoses 'hysteria' and she calms down; she's grateful. My wife and I laugh out loud at the screen: you'd be jailed for doing that now. Cronin, Céline and Bulgakov: throw them all in the slammer!

And it's so good to hear Bulgakov complaining about poor referral letters. I'd like to show him some of the ones I got. How about this:

Dear Doctor,
This man has anal pain. Please see and advise.
   Yrs

Succinct, you can say that for it. This was on the back of a used Benson & Hedges pack. And then I read this from Bulgakov's story 'The Blizzard': 'I felt the customary cold in the pit of my stomach, as I always did when I saw death close to. I hate death.'

Don't we all, mate, don't we all.

17

WOBBLERS

You have to hate death to be a doctor, and fear that cold in the pit, that freezing point that insists on action: action now, before it's too late. Bulgakov's 'customary' is the right word. The chill in the stomach is instantaneous, inescapable.

Here's another night tale.

Brighton, one in the morning, and I get a call from the registrar. We spoke a couple of hours ago, before I fell asleep, and all was well. That was before Anne arrived. The registrar tells me she is eighteen and very ill. She is near comatose and pyrexial, feverish. Her neck is as stiff as a board and she has a rash. He's sure she has bacterial meningitis and has given her a whack of antibiotics and arranged for her to go to ITU. I tell him I'll be there in ten minutes and get out of bed and head out into the rain. The wind is blowing hard from the east. The roads are empty, there's not another soul walking the streets, no lights on in the seafront houses. The odd lonely seagull squawks.

Six years ago I was told a similar story and by the time I made it up to A+E, fifteen minutes from bed to ward, the young man was dead. Bacterial meningitis. Dead despite being given antibiotics. Every doctor on the planet fears bacterial meningitis.

Anne is lying on her bed in ITU, her hair in wet strands over her damp forehead as if she's been pulled out of the water; she looks like Everett Millais' limp Ophelia. Her mouth hangs slackly open and her pulse is thready; her blood pressure needs inotropic support with infusions of noradrenaline. The only positive is that she is so ill she is not in pain; she lies there 'incapable of her own distress'.

Looking down at Anne, I'm immediately reminded of another patient, a young Jamaican girl we admitted a few years back and how we struggled to save her. She too was not yet twenty years old. She died of sudden fulminant sepsis within an hour of arrival, again despite antibiotics and inotropes. At post-mortem the pathologists could not find a spleen. She had been born without one. You need a spleen to fight infection. Sometimes sickle-cell anaemia can cause splenic infarction, but we'd thought of that and checked her for sickle on arrival. She did not have sickle: she simply but disastrously had no spleen. All her life she had been a walking time bomb but didn't know it. Tragically she was always going to die if and when she caught pneumococcal sepsis. She was very, very unlucky. People who have their spleen removed after an accident receive prophylaxis against pneumococcal infection. She would have too if it had been known she'd been born without a spleen, but how was anyone to guess that?

The idea of walking around with some occult, internal sword of Damocles is frightening. Yet one might argue we all do, it's just that it falls sooner on the heads of some.

Anne on ITU is now under another consultant. But as she arrived during my time on call she will return to my ward if she's lucky enough to pull through. If she were to die I'd be called to the coroner's court. They would rightly ask had I confirmed the management plan and had I seen her. Not long before, in another hospital, a consultant had not gone in to see a man who died as he waited to be transferred to a specialist unit. The tabloid newspapers labelled him Dr Do Little.

I go in to double-check the care plan and to see her parents, to talk to them, to try to deal with their fears. They sit beside her and occasionally lean over and wipe her brow, Dad at one side, Mum on the other. Anne's little sister is also in the room and she sobs quietly in a corner chair. Both parents stare down helplessly at their gravely ill daughter. I ask if I can speak to them together and we move to a quiet room where I explain the diagnosis. The father asks: 'Is that why she has that rash?'

'Yes.'

Dad seems a gentle man. His words are slow and deliberate, his manner calm, resigned. It strikes me quickly that he may be in an allied profession: his eyes, in some mysterious way, express an understanding of my explanations, my occasional lapse into jargon. He remains unfazed as I utter words like 'inotrope'. He tells me he's a radiographer and so he knows our language, knows what it implies. I take a deep breath: 'I'm afraid Anne is very sick.'

'I know.'

'We'll have a better idea of which way things are going by dawn.'

We share a few more words together and then I accompany them back to the unit and Anne's bed. There's nothing more to do just now except urge them to hang on in there.

Hang on in there. See you in the morning. And then I think: I really need to get out of the habit of saying these trite phrases. I've got to come up with a better word than 'hang'.

When I arrive back on ITU after a couple of hours' kip Anne is still alive, her blood pressure up. The team is more confident. I speak with Dad again. He sighs with relief when I say she's going to make it. Then he breaks: 'This is so awful.'

'I understand.'

We say this a lot. *I understand*. And yet we don't. Not really. How could we? If this hasn't happened to you, a daughter with bacterial meningitis, how can you *really* understand?

But maybe there's a chink. You've got to use your imagination, try on unthinkable thoughts. If you are a reader, if you have marinated yourself in novels and tried to imagine what it must be like to have someone else's problems, to be in someone else's world, then maybe, just maybe, you might get a glimpse of understanding.

Two weeks later Anne leaves the hospital; she does not need to see me professionally again. Her dad asks me a couple of months later if I would like to go to a concert with them to celebrate her recovery and I go along and have a fine evening. Now, ten years later, I still see them socially. She has a great job and a great partner. She's alive.

Her father called last week to tell me that Anne is now pregnant. He's going to be a grandfather. I want to see this baby when he or she arrives.

I'm asked to go to court and be a defence witness for one of my patients. He's a rogue but he's not an evil man, more the feckless sort; there is no shortage of those in this life. Ron has diabetes and he sometimes takes his insulin, sometimes not. He's uncertain how to give the correct doses but then many young doctors who prescribe the stuff aren't that sure either. I get his case notes out and confirm his irregular attendance at the clinic, his poor control, his frequent episodes of hypoglycaemia. He's been arrested for causing a disturbance of the peace. Ron has been verbally abusive to the arresting officer, threatening him with violence and so on. The police allege he was drunk. Ron says he was hypoglycaemic. *Failure to induce hypoglycaemia in Glaswegian alcoholics.* But Ron isn't an alcoholic. Or Glaswegian. He's from Hove, actually. Who's telling the truth? That's what the court is set to decide. I'm called to the box. The defence lawyer begins to question me: 'Is it possible that my client was hypoglycaemic? Is it possible he had a low blood sugar [here she nods in explanation to the judge] the night he was arrested?'

'It is.'

I explain to the judge (I was taught: *always* address the judge) how hypoglycaemia can cause behavioural change, how this can mimic inebriation due to alcohol, how it can be corrected by ingestion of glucose. The defence continues: 'Can we exclude the possibility that my client was hypoglycaemic?'

'No. I don't think we can.'

The defence lawyer sits and it is now the turn of the prosecution. I recall my training in legal medicine, the courses I've been on. Look and talk to the judge. Listen to the questions but do not look at the prosecutor. On the course they told us (with some force) that the lawyers hold all the cards. They can undermine you before you've said a single word. If you are *not* an academic they might deliberately address you as 'Professor' before a swift verbal redaction and then adding: 'Ah, of course but you are not a professor, are you?'

Job done.

And even if you *are* an academic, even if you are the most famous professor in your chosen specialty on the planet, they can introduce you politely, deferentially, and then say something like: 'We are now in April, Professor, April being the cruellest month as I'm sure you know. Just how many international conferences have you addressed this year, Professor? Wait, I see from my records once a month so far: Auckland, Chicago, Tokyo, mmmm Rio. And examining for your college in Dubai, that doesn't leave a lot of time for seeing actual real live patients, does it, Professor? How many have you actually *seen* this year, six or seven maybe?'

So they've got you before you even open your mouth. Mind you, at least they don't ask if I'm related to Dr Quinn, medicine woman.

The prosecution begins: 'How can you be sure that Ron was hypoglycaemic rather than drunk on the night in question?'

'I can't. But there is a way we could have been.'

'Oh yes? And what might that be?'

'He could have had a blood sugar reading done. A simple stick test.'

The prosecution team ruffle their notes noisily. Nobody checked Ron's blood sugar and so hypoglycaemia could not be excluded as a cause for his outbursts. And so Ron is cleared.

Two months later I'm told that Ron is dead. He died shortly after his release. Fell and cut his leg and bled to death. I can't help but wonder if he would have been safer in prison. And I'll never know if he was actually hypoglycaemic that night he swore at the cops or if he was just drunk. We will never know either if he was hypoglycaemic the night he cut an artery. Medicine is full of these ironies, these mysteries, these what-ifs.

I've been meaning to submit a scenario to the Royal College of Physicians for a possible test of communication skills in the PACES exam. I wonder how candidates would deal with a situation I've come across with increasing frequency in my last few years of working. An old man enters the clinic room to discuss his diabetes control.

'How much insulin are you currently taking?'

'Come again?'

'How much...?'

And here I'd point to the plastic bag he's plonked on my desk with its pens and meters and jotters. Those jotters where he's scribbled his blood tests and/or smeared blood on the pages. He'd work out what I was getting at: 'Oh, whatever I think is right.'

Not a good start. I'd noted his unsteady gait as he walked into the clinic room. Noticed too his mild tremor, maybe he has early Parkinson's. Should I mention that?

'Have you had any hypos?'

'Pardon?'

'Hypos, you know: low blood sugars, blood sugars under four?'

Four is the floor. The new message from the British Diabetes Association, our new mantra: kinda catchy.

'I've had the odd wobbler, yes. Nothing I can't handle.'

Wobbler. He wobbles like a child's toy. Like a Weeble, the old boy wobbles but he doesn't fall down. He tells me he still gets to Glyndebourne with all the other Weebles. (He doesn't say that last bit.) He likes his opera. I'm going through the computer records of his care and now typing in his last blood tests; his diabetes control is indifferent. I'm not too bothered about that as I don't particularly *want* him to have tight control: he's in his mid-eighties and he's more at risk of hypos and falling if we try too hard to get normoglycaemia. I come to the section on his records that specifically relates to driving: 'You're not still driving, are you?'

'I am. Problem with that?'

He's heard that one all right. He's leaning forward now, staring at me. I pause: 'Well...'

I click on to the next few screens and look at his cardiovascular risk calculator: the percentage risk estimate of this man having a significant cardiovascular event in the next year. A stroke. A heart attack. A high figure is now screaming out at me. If you were motoring quite merrily of a Sunday afternoon and you knew that the man in the car on the other lane, approaching you at 70 mph, had a near 100 per cent chance of a stroke in the next year I suspect you too would be very frightened. I tell him I don't think it's a good idea for him to continue driving. He explodes: 'WHAT? I need my car! I need my car to get food for my wife, you of all people know how sick she is!'

He reminds me that he lives in the countryside. The nearest shops are two miles away. He can't walk there and back. He sits back in his chair now, his manner exasperated, annoyed. He doesn't like me any more, if he ever did. I try to explain to him the risk calculations, but he doesn't want to know *that* percentage when I tell him I have it on the screen before me. Well, would you? It's as near as we get to giving someone an expiry date. And that's something most of us don't really want to hear: you're good before 2041.

I try another tactic: 'Look, you've got a terrific life. You've got your wife, your family. You see your *Così fan tutte*. You can look back on your life too and smile, I hope. But listen, let's just imagine you had a prang and it was because your blood sugar was low. You wouldn't forgive yourself, would you?'

He's silent, looking at me sullenly. I go on: 'And what if you were unlucky enough to hit someone else? They might seek compensation. You don't want that. And if you're really unlucky you might hurt them or even kill them! That might mean being charged with manslaughter. You could even be sent to jail.'

'Oh, come on now, Doctor, don't be so dramatic!'

He makes a sweeping gesture with his arms and struggles to get up. After maybe another thirty minutes of careful explanation he leaves, now resolved, so he tells me, to sell his car. I've convinced him. If we used this scenario in the exam, in PACES, you would have had twelve minutes to get to this conclusion.

Real life: I'm looking at a picture of a young girl with brown hair and blue eyes, brilliantly white teeth set in a beaming smile. Her eyeliner is subtly done, her face gleams with youth and beauty. Then I read this:

> An elderly driver has been found guilty of causing the death of a teenage girl in a horror crash on a petrol station forecourt. Alexander Wotherspoon, eighty-three, killed seventeen-year-old Eilish Herron when he reversed into her at speed as she filled her car at the Asda petrol station in Linwood, Renfrewshire.

Linwood, not far from where we once lived in Glasgow. The jury, I read, took just over an hour to convict him.

A gap between patients and I wash my hands. How many times a day do I wash my hands? The hand gel dispenser below the sink mirror ejaculates over my shirt. That's just great. And now the coiled cords of my landline and my computer have managed to tie themselves together: how do they do that? The wires copulate as incessantly as a pair of intestinal worms. I hate these fucking wires as much as I would a personal infestation of such creatures. I try to untangle them but by the end of the afternoon they're back encoiled in congress. Then I can't open the window. The room is boiling: it's high summer but the hospital heating is still on. I can't open the window because a painter has coated the wood outside and thus it's now jammed shut. Worse, the roller blind keeps jumping its teeth and I have to clamber up onto my desk and stretch up to fix the little plastic ball things back in place. The phone rings when I'm up there, the phone rings if I get up for a slash and then stops when I scramble back into the room to answer it. Returning from the loo, I look at the emails: yet another survey to fill in, this time from the RCP. At what age are you planning retirement? *Right now.*

The year passes and it is winter again; some drifts of snow have closed down the south of England. Colleagues are snowbound. They live on the other side of the Downs. I've got to cover. The whole system has frozen up, it's going to hell, a frozen hell like that weird infernal world Dante talks about.

Medicine gets harder as you age. This is not so much due to fatigue, or a Timon of Athens-like creeping misanthropy, but perhaps because it becomes less funny. The laughs come harder, the jokes take on a darker edge; all that's left is a form of gallows humour. *We're all gonna die.* A lame form of satire: the province of the fool waving his pig-bladder, the jester with his bitter sneers; an unappealing sight. And irony, as Czesław Miłosz once said, 'Irony is the glory of slaves.'

Here's an ironic story.

One of my Deanery duties is to visit other hospitals and report on training: in the parlance, this is 'educational governance'. I'm visiting the other side of our patch. The local head of the education department, an oncologist, is close to tears as she tells me about a difficult colleague. She tells me this man's manner is persistently disdainful; he's not a team player. His colleagues report that he is not skilled in communicating with immigrants or the disadvantaged or the uneducated. The words 'not skilled' are a euphemism. His absences grow more frequent: he's said to be at the college or at a conference or God knows where. Senior management is aware of concerns as regards his infrequent presence. She tells me about complaints from patients and other colleagues; these mount up. She tells me she has spoken to her medical director. The oncologist dabs at her eyes. It's my job to probe: 'So what does the medical director say?'

She calms herself: 'The MD?'

Taking a deep breath, she's careful with her next remarks: 'He doesn't specify exactly *why* he can't hold our colleague to account. My suspicion is that he doesn't want to open a can of worms.'

'A can of worms?'

Then there's a silence. I break it: 'Might that can have something to do with the private sector. A conflict of interest?'

My mind flashes back to A. J. Cronin's *The Citadel* and the character Dr Manson with his own, similar, ethical challenges to do with the private sector. Cronin published the novel in 1937. More than eighty years have passed since its publication and we've still got the same old same old. The silence of the oncologist suggests that maybe some of her other colleagues would end up under investigation if that can were opened and yada yada yah. She says that she has had to put up with a decade of such managerial prevarication. NHS 'whistle-blowers' are sent to various versions of Coventry, various forms of Siberia.

Towards the end of my involvement in this saga the Associate Deans are told they are to have a prolonged appraisal as part of new national procedures. Seventy sections have to be completed online. After submission I meet with the Dean's deputy. In standard fashion he initially relays some finessed praise but then gives me the 'constructive feedback': 'You have difficulty holding some people to account.'

At last we get the *real* diagnosis: this is what really ails the NHS. *We have difficulty holding some people to account.* No, make that the political problem in general: our global political diagnosis. We can't hold the powerful to account.

Irony is the glory of slaves.

18

TO THE FRENCH HOUSE, THAT'S THE WAY

'Write as much as you possibly can!'

So says Chekhov in a letter to Maria Kiselyova. He goes on: 'Initially at least a good half of your stuff will be sent back to you accompanied by a rejection slip… Don't let it upset you.'

I keep pitching. I'm getting more reviews published. *ArtReview* have asked me to go to Istanbul again; they've accepted work from Vienna, Berlin, Buenos Aires and Glasgow. I chat with Andrew O'Hagan after one of his readings and he listens to the outline of a novel I've written: he's encouraging and gives me his agent's details. I meet her a month later in Soho and she's politely interested too. After seven years at the Deanery on Tooley Street I make up my mind: it's time to move on. Those Fridays are for writing now. The hospital managers agree that I can work ten hours a day Monday to Thursday and only do Fridays when the rota says I'm on call or due to cover the wards.

So I'm down to a putative forty-hour week now that I'm in my early fifties. While doing appraisals I'm struck by how many consultant colleagues have a long-term agreement that seems to allow them a day a week free for private work. I insist on this new Friday arrangement because, after nearly thirty years of service, it's my turn to have a similarly flexible work pattern. I should have suggested this years before. Mug.

My concern for the service nationally intensifies and I decide to stand in an RCP election seeking new council members. My blurb, in part, parodies the usual bumf submitted by prospective candidates. Fuckin' comedian. These blurbs, these adverts, usually take the form of a mini-CV that outlines the number of committees a prospective candidate has sat on. This number is usually quite large. The candidate usually omits saying that this burden conveniently excuses them from overt clinical work, the front line.

The college asks for a photograph to go along with the voting papers. I decide against the usual 'you can trust me' shot: the suit and tie, the car salesman smile, the head tilted ever so slightly to imply that you really, really care. *Always give it the caring jazz.* I have mine taken looking upwards as if I'm in deep existential despair. I remember that falling couple in the print I disliked. I'm not one for allegory but that couple now seems emblematic of the fall: the decline of the NHS. My photograph tries to hint to the voter: *Hey, although I've tried to write something funny here I'm actually quite a serious guy. The problems we now face are really desperate, right?* Perhaps this scepticism rings a bell with the electorate; I'm voted on. The first time I've had the guts to stand for anything.

The council meets in the RCP building across from Regent's Park in a modernist cube designed by Denys Lasdun. The council chambers are a chalk-white circular space that bears a distinct resemblance to the War Room in Kubrick's *Dr Strangelove*. The president sits at twelve o'clock and we, the council, sit along the circumference and raise points of order. When I contribute, I do my best to avoid coming across like the gum-chewing jingoist General Buck Turgidson, as played by George C. Scott. There are quite a few turgid matters for discussion, though. Then the president resets the tone, gets down to proper business.

The discussions get heavier and heavier. What is our line on euthanasia? Do we give the position document our approval? The next item revolves around a recent manslaughter case. New plans for specialty training are being developed with a renewed focus on generalist skills. We are becoming too American in our approach: patients are getting too many specialist opinions without one doctor overseeing the big picture. We are back to Kalanithi's question about WICOS: who is the captain of the ship? Here I fight my specialty's corner; endocrinologists exceed generalist expectations by some way. Registrars in endocrinology seem to do much more of the general medical take, as opposed to, say, cardiologists, rheumatologists, neurologists: hence our difficulty in recruitment.

The medical registrar, not to put too fine a point on it, is *dumped* on. Bow-tied neurologists attract my ire because you'll rarely see any of them down in A+E. Get them down there seeing poorly controlled epilepsy, the frozen Parkinsonian. Covid-19 should change the abuse of the medical registrar for ever… but will it? We await a reconfiguration of roles.

Back in the War Room we go on to discuss the RCP response to strike action by our junior colleagues. A belligerent Health Secretary is dead set against the juniors and their demands.

The juniors duly strike. We seniors act down. I am the only doctor available for our ward of twenty inpatients. I pick old ladies off the floor. I write up prescriptions and discharge letters. Put in request forms. All good fun in a nostalgic kind of way, but this is bad, very bad practice. Bad for patients. I can't do all this routine stuff *and* think clearly about major decisions – *Should this person be tube-fed? Should this other be for resuscitation?* – this is asking too much. Putting the generals on the front line is a desperate move. Trust is ebbing away; the juniors are talking of leaving for New Zealand and Australia. Oz with its xenophobic taxi drivers and transphobic cardinals. That can't be right.

The college earns enough money from its exams to hold an annual dinner in honour of William Harvey and his circulatory discoveries as per those drawings I saw at Eton. Tonight's key speaker is the head of the NHS. He spars with the president at speech time. We are served water buffalo. The thin slices are succulent. A waiter squirts some perfume over our heads as we eat. Scent from the veldt, we're told.

The man to my right is elderly, distinguished, a dandy; he wears medals. I think about quoting to him Murat's line that he wore medals 'so that people will shoot at me' but don't. He has a naval bearing, but I decide it's maybe best not to talk about past wars. Turns out he is the boss of the Jerwood Foundation. We spend the evening (bizarrely) discussing Jake and Dinos Chapman's recent show at the Jerwood's gallery in Hastings. He is unflappable; the brothers and their use of ectopic penises do not shock him. He's probably seen many atrocious things in real life. He admits their work is not his cup of tea. Why is he here? He tells me that he advises the college on wine. He raises his glass and asks me: 'What do you think of this one, then?'

'Tastes fine to me.'

'Bit weak.'

'You know your wine. You're an oenophile.'

I feel weirdly pressurised into using the word, a plea, in effect, that asks him to believe that I've had *some* education. He expands: 'Yes. I spent many years in Portugal.'

'Aha. Working as?'

'I was the chief executive of Dow's. You know, the port?'

I'm spending an inordinate amount of time with the bosses of major alcohol concerns these days: this is not on message as regards RCP statements about the stuff.

After two years on council I'm asked to appraise the president. We meet in her office. She is doing her best in very trying circumstances. Her reasoned, tranquil manner seems appropriately rational in the teeth of these politically bullying times. As I sit with her, I realise that this is a final high of my career in medicine. I think, but do not say, that we cannot win against the current mood of the people. That she, and we, will not win. That the people are voting against proper funding, against a proper future for the NHS. All political careers end in failure, as has been said all too often. It's downhill all the way from here. As Private Frazer would say in *Dad's Army*: *We're doomed!*

When it comes to summing up the appraisal, I'm like the decrepit old department store owner in yet another British TV sitcom, *Are You Being Served?* I'm like the ancient codger wheeled out in his chair at the end of the show. As he leaves with his nurse, the crinkly old buffer waves his walking stick and shouts: *You're all doing very well!*

'To the French House, that's the way': this is a line from a terrific song by an obscure (albeit excellent, now defunct) band from

Edinburgh called the Nectarine Number Nine, another Davy Henderson project. They're now reborn with an even better name: The Sexual Objects. I find myself singing those lines every time I'm up in Soho and pass the French House. The French with its flags waving outside, the tricolor, and that other blue one bearing the fleur-de-lis. The French has become an irregular stopping-off point on my travels in London. They don't serve beer by the cask, I'm not even sure if they sell *any* beer, and the wine… well, let's just say the wine tastes of wine. One day, back down in Brighton, I call in the next patient, a man called Collins, who runs the French House.

Collins is another cheery Falstaffian endomorph with Type 2 diabetes. He's clearly a bon viveur. When I ask about his alcohol intake he tells me he can get through a couple of bottles of Chablis. I press him: 'A week?'

He chokes with suppressed mirth: 'A *week*? God, no! I mean a day, man! Over a fine lunch!'

We go through the routine questioning, but he is quick to inveigle some concessions to his lifestyle. 'Inveigle' is the operative word here. Collins is a cajoler, a coaxer, a wheedler, a persuader. Or should I say a 'Persuader'? I now see Collins as a composite figure: one-part Roger Moore with his patrician Dulwich College accent, his vowels occasionally chewed, as if chomping on a treacle and butter toffee from Fortnum & Mason. His other half would be Tony Curtis with his cheeky self-confidence, that glint in his eye that warns you, like Mark Twain again, he will not let the truth get in the way of a good story. Collins was a journalist and loves tall tales; his boyish enthusiasm for a yarn is catching; he is Tom Sawyer grown up, Tom in the flesh. In turn I become Huck, his slow-witted pal, as I listen to his stories and try to keep up.

Collins's arteries are as furred up as a Sussex chalk-encrusted kettle. He limps painfully. I have to see him regularly: 'What are you working on now?'

'I'm nearly finished with my Diana book.'

'Oh yeah? You're not going to tell me she was murdered, are you?'

'Of course I am! Of course she was!'

'Oh, get away with you.'

'She was, I'm telling you, John. I've heard it from [he leans in now and winks slowly] let's say highly informed sources.'

I'm killing myself with laughter: 'Who? Langley?'

'Now, now, John. But you're on the right track. She was taken out because of her stance on land mines. Fact.'

'But wasn't it something to do with a little white car? That Fiat Uno?'

Collins ignores my cheek and tells me about James Andanson, paparazzi photographer and informer for MI6; how he was later found dead in a burnt-out car. The Friends again. Collins knows a worrying amount about Diana's death. I try to surprise him by saying: 'Hey, we were also in Paris that night.'

Fact.

Just after midnight we were in a cab driving south from the Pigalle to the Rue du Bac. My wife and I had been refused entry into a dance hall because we were too uncool. I tell him maybe in our frustration *we* accidentally killed her.

Collins wags a finger at me. He's not in the mood today to talk about his other books, his compilations of obscure facts. He's on serious reporter mode and now dips his head and speaks quietly, more slowly: *She was murdered, John.*

Collins makes me think again about Graham Greene: Greene in Sierra Leone. I've often wondered: what was Greeneland, what do the people said to inhabit that mythical place look like? I imagine some of them must have been like Collins. Silver-haired, shirt a tad crumpled, with a yellow and red striped silk MCC tie around his neck (was he *really* a member?). I'm looking at a photograph of him raising a glass and he is indeed wearing one of the raffish jackets the MCC favoured. Raffish; Collins was raffish. Did he work for The Friends? Who knows? Maybe he knew Ross McKenzie, my old boss up in Stirling. Maybe they hung out together in Paraguay or Yemen.

He would bring me copies of his books: many of these lined the wall behind the gantry at the French House. Collins had worked for the *News of the World* and so knew alcohol was a truth drug. Collins told me that he had set up the AAA (the Anti-Alcoholics Anonymous), a group that would do its best to dissuade anyone from teetotalism. He tells me stories about Francis Bacon and Dan Farson and Jeffrey Bernard and Keith Waterhouse: *He lived in Brighton too, you know, in one of those top flats at Embassy Court.* Lamely I mention that Nabokov loved *Jubb*, a novel by Waterhouse, the follow-up to *Billy Liar*. Collins isn't interested in that; he wants to tell me about his new pal: Suggs from Madness. *Suggs, you know, 'One Step Beyond', lovely man, very clever too.*

Collins is a member of the Groucho. I tell him we once blagged a trip to the club with some artists and saw Neil the Pet Shop Boy in a corner. A man from Beck's beer signed us in. Later he asked if I wanted some cocaine. I was polite: no, thank you. Collins loves all this nonsense. He tells me salacious stories about Hughie Green and Paula Yates, about Princess Margaret, about Juan Perón, who he says he knew in Madrid. Collins wanted me to sign up for the AAA. I declined, citing my college responsibilities.

Collins wrote Shockingly Frank and Revealing Accounts for the

Sunday papers; he was proud to be a fount of useless information; his Elvis impression was a hoot. Better than mine, that's for sure.

I read a few months after my retirement that Collins died suddenly while nursing a glass of champagne. In the *Guardian* obituary Roy Greenslade repeated a taunt Collins was fond of quoting, a literary warning I'd do well to remember, a Mark Twain jibe about Henry James: 'Once you've put one of his books down, you simply can't pick it up again.'

19

FIRST HE GIVES US DIAMONDS

I look at myself in the bathroom mirror this morning. I'm getting older. Everyone is getting older. Last night I watched an ancient BBC production of *Titus Andronicus*. Titus asks his brother to look at his face. *Witness these trenches made by grief and care.* I stare again at my own frown lines. We're in a new decade, it's 2010, and I'm frowning constantly at the deliberate political undermining of the NHS. I've been frowning so much that I've got a trench face like Titus. I'd been worried about turning into another Shakespearean sad-sack: Timon. Timon, the Athenian who tired of dishing out diamonds as gifts. Disappointed, he now gave ordinary pebbles as presents to his fair-weather friends. I'm not Timon, not yet. Maybe I'm Titus Face. Maybe I'm getting like Titus: thrashing around in my own grief and care.

The complaints department are on the phone about a man who died six months or so ago. I'm shocked and saddened to learn only now that the man had died.

I get the notes out and see that I met the patient one extremely busy Saturday afternoon. He was in his late seventies and had significant comorbidities. We arranged for his transfer to another team that afternoon. In the early hours he arrested.

We made a wrong diagnostic call. We did everything else: admitted the man, gave him analgesia, kept him comfortable, but... we got it wrong.

We apologise unreservedly. A later independent report concludes: 'It is highly likely that the patient would have still died from the condition.' Would have died. Still died. Highly likely. *Highly* likely.

There are recommendations that the organisation publicise the case to prevent repetition; that lessons be learned. This we do. I deliver the take-home message at a grand round, my last ever. This would be the exact inverse of my first presentation, that prior success I had as a house officer, now more than thirty years ago. The bottle of anchovy sauce and the slice of bread, the belly laughs as I poured. But this is now, and this is the twenty-first century, this is where I beat my breast in front of my peers. This is my public mea culpa, mea maxima culpa.

I have had annual appraisals and never known anything of a punitive nature: I've even known a degree of praise. I have tried to do my very best. Look, I want to plead, I want to shout: I, we, didn't do it deliberately! I, we, made a mistake, a simple mistake. Don't we all make mistakes?

The day in question was extremely busy. Another bed crisis. Phones going off everywhere. Mayhem. Patients piling in. Pandemonium. The receiving ward, the so-called Medical Assessment Unit, was in bedlam. An excuse, I know, but a very real one, one that all hospital doctors will recognise.

The patient got care, free at the point of delivery. We will *always* get something wrong in medicine: this does not mean a failure *of* care implies a failure *to* care. There are more mistakes made daily than most of the public would care to know about. Humans make mistakes, especially if we are working with fewer resources. And in particular if we try to deliver care under austerity measures with patients stacked in corridors.

Failure is irritating, that's obvious. Failure *hurts*. And I get irked (not again!) with another literary great and what he had to say about failure. That Beckett 'fail better' quote from *Worstward Ho* crops up in reviews and articles almost weekly. Failure: as for that novel I had hopes for, I hear no more from the agent in Soho.

Dispirited, I wonder about chucking out my copy of James Knowlson's Beckett biography. Maybe I should give it to the Marie Curie shop. Hand it in for the sick, the dying. There's black humour for you, there's being a fuckin' comedian. Imagine finding a second-hand copy of Beckett in a charity shop that supports a hospice. Even worse: imagine being in a hospice; imagine actively dying and reading Beckett's famous lines. Fuck it: here they are one more time.

Ever tried. Ever failed. No matter. Try again. Fail again. Fail better.

But you can't. Not in the NHS. You can't fail better any more working in the NHS now. Not under the current conditions. Not with underfunding. Was Beckett just trying to make us *feel* a little bit better? No. Beckett wasn't a doctor. That's what we do: try to make people feel better. Even if they're poggered.

Then the deaths began: the deaths of colleagues, five in five months. Their deaths and what they taught me.

The first to die was Gregor. I didn't know him. This is something of his story as I heard it. One day he was asked to help with a patient needing a nasogastric tube. In the process of insertion the patient became distressed. Senior types duly arrived and called the police. They in turn arrested Gregor. He was suspended. The case went to court many months later. The judge threw it out, but the damage had been done.

Gregor had been exonerated. Many colleagues testified that he was an exceptionally kind and caring man. They also hinted that he had been treated with great shabbiness. A few weeks after the verdict he hooked himself up to an infusion of high-dosage sedation and let the drug do its worst.

Two months later I'm sipping on a coffee in the canteen and one of the professors comes up to me: had I heard the news? He tells me the story and I hear him and then swear under my breath. And then stare blankly out at the flat sea.

Martin Fisher was appointed just after me, twenty or more years ago. When he arrived, our patients with HIV were dying at a ludicrous rate. With the advent of the protease inhibitor drugs, Martin and his team began to save lives. He built up a unit that was now internationally renowned. He published widely, appointed more and more members to his team. I'd meet him for the odd pint in Kemptown and he'd tell me about his recent holiday trip on the Trans-Siberian; what he had been listening to recently; about his renewed optimism for the future of HIV medicine.

I was a little envious of the excitement in his specialty: mine was somewhat stuck in a rut after a sequence of serious advances in the 1980s. His fortieth birthday party was held in the aquarium near the pier. He did some DJing. He liked house music and Bowie. He was made professor. At fifty he was at the peak of his career.

Many of the members of the local gay community were at his memorial. Some stood and spoke out about his generosity of spirit, how he had saved their lives, how he had kept them going during the dark days before the new drugs. A straight couple with HIV also told of their concern when the woman fell pregnant, of how Martin had cared brilliantly for them and how the baby was fine.

A wonderfully brave refugee, an African woman, talked of how Martin had fought the Home Office to ensure that she was given life-saving treatment. She reminded us that few are so lucky.

Martin's photograph was projected on a screen. He was one of those doctors with a kind of imploring look that asked: *Believe me, I can help you.* I imagine he was probably asked for directions in the street all the time, questioned as to where the bread was kept when he ventured into Asda or Marks & Spencer's. They played Bowie's 'Heroes' at the end of the service. The Martin Fisher Foundation, formed in 2015, remembers him and continues his work towards zero HIV infections, zero HIV-related deaths. Give them your support.

A week later and I get a call from Manchester. My patient Aidan has died. Aidan had been chief medical officer in Ireland and then worked in the UK as a professor. I met him first when he had been seconded to our hospital to advise on safety. He gave me a grilling about a man who had died from overwhelming sepsis and who had diabetes. We agreed that some processes involving communication with the surgeons could be improved. Aidan was a fan of Atul Gawande and his checklists. I was impressed by Aidan's focus; his desire to make systems work better and save lives. Then he himself developed diabetes. His control was not as good as he, or I, would have wished, but he was one of those people, invariably successful, who would park his own health concerns and expend all his energy on the wellbeing of others. Maybe this was a form of denial. We spoke about this at our long sessions when I would see him at the end of a clinic. Inevitably we would get on to politics. He was never despondent about the free market challenges he faced as a public health doctor. He fought tirelessly at the Department of Health for a better deal for the homeless. He knew his fight for the homeless was just.

As a Dubliner, he knew his Joyce and Beckett; he was supportive of my literary delusions. We would shake hands at the end of each consultation after I'd recommended a novel to him and he a recent polemical tract to me. I can hear him now: he talked to me like a big brother to his younger, dafter, sibling: 'You're a good lad.'

Maybe that's all we really want to hear as doctors. Encouragements, restrained praise, a bit of affection. Doctors *love* love. We are greedy for love. Many doctors I've known are fortunate enough to have been brought up by loving parents, they often have great relationships with their own brothers or sisters, but somehow that's not enough. Maybe there is no such thing as enough love. Doctors like being doctors because they get more love. We might as well face it. Doctors in part become doctors because... they're addicted to love.

I can't remember how many times I told Aidan to stop smoking, to take some time out on holiday, to be more selfish, to look after himself, but he would wave me off with a 'sure, I will, don't worry' and then come back to see me a few months later and shiftily, shyly, admit that he was still having the odd puff. We are deprived of a dedicated, good man, a man who knew his Orwell, who knew that those poor down-and-outs in Brighton and London were worthy of our time, our care and our humanity.

And then there was number four, Frank, a locum consultant who would arrive for the morning handover looking permanently exhausted. Maybe he was hungover. He looked like a man who enjoyed life to the full. And then one morning he was found in his office. Another cardiovascular event.

People said things like: 'Well, he was a smoker.' This is what medics do with death. Try to rationalise it. They can imply (some might say callously) that it was all his or her own fault. If only he or she had stopped drinking/smoking/loafing and started exercising.

Maybe it might not have happened. There is an all-pervasive rush to judge in medicine, in public life in general these days. One minute you're here; the next, gone. The world shrugs and says: 'Well, that was tough luck.' That's your lot. Summed up and quickly forgotten. No room for sympathy. Confronted with sad news, my dad would quote a daffy sports commentator he loved called Syd Waddell: 'There's no room for sympathy in full-time darts.'

Lastly there was Charles. Charles was one of the juniors I was most proud to help train. He'd only recently been appointed as a consultant to his home island of Barbados. Charles reminded me, in his movement and gestures, of the great fast bowler Michael Holding. He'd carry a slim briefcase on his ward rounds. He was as graceful in his bedside manner as Michael was with his cheetah-like run-up. Charles developed leukaemia and didn't make forty. I can't square what I remember of him with this fact.

Five deaths in five months. And here I am sitting at my desk getting fatter. I'm going home and stuffing my face with grilled coconut prawns and spag bol and something profoundly atherogenic from Marks & Spencer's called a 'billionaire's dessert', a chocolate and caramel sweet-covered creation with tacky gold flakes, and we're downing a bottle of Californian Pinot Noir. This can't go on.

So we book a flight to see my uncles in Vancouver for some healthy living and soon we're with one of them, Dan (Aunt June's brother), as he tugs at his oxygen mask and his heavy gas canisters that gamely try to counter his pulmonary hypertension. Like his sister June he has big cardiac problems. We splash out and dine downtown at one of Dan's old stomping grounds before his ill health struck, a place called Hawksworth. We hit on the seared Japanese squid done with peanuts, nashi pear and crispy pork chilli vinaigrette as an appetiser; entrées of caramelised scallops, pan-roasted lingcod and halibut tempura. More Pinot Noir is drunk, this time from the Okanagan Valley. I raise a glass to the ladies, my aunt, my mum and my wife. My two uncles josh about the upcoming Canadian election. Dan, somehow maintaining his jollity despite the oxygen prongs, is a Trudeau man and wants his old liberal country back. My other uncle, Nick, is sober, restrained, wants more time with the Conservatives. My mum enjoys her seafood: she's happy to be here with her wee brother, her big sister. We head onto West Georgia Street planning to drive out to White Rock near the US border. White Rock with its views of the Pacific, its wee pier reminding them of home, its big white boulder (hence the name), where they all live now in peace and quiet, away from the inner city and its madness. We cross the concourse of an HSBC towards the underground car park and my mum turns to me and says: 'I feel...'

She barfs copiously, frighteningly, suddenly, onto the polished marble of the bank's flooring. Everyone turns to stare at us. Dan puts his oxygen tank down and we both support my mum and somehow get her into the lobby of the Rosewood hotel. The Rosewood runs Hawksworth.

The manager, initially, is not particularly helpful, but his tone changes when he learns of Dan's past employment history as an insurer and my suspicion that mum has scombroid poisoning. 'That's scombroid: ess, sea, oh, ehm, bee, ahr, oh, aye, dee. You get it with fish gone off. I suspect this might be the diagnosis. I'm a physician.' The manager is not impressed at first; maybe he thinks I'm a conman. We endure a lecture about the freshness of the fish and the necessity of getting an ambulance, but I'm sure what my mum needs right now is just a lie-down somewhere. The manager concedes and gets us a room. Mum slowly recovers without us spending a fortune in a Vancouver hospital.

I'm fried. Once we get home to the UK, I hear that Uncle Nick has had a fit. Nick gets an MRI scan and then is told he has a grade four glioblastoma, the very worst type of brain tumour. Grade four: Stevenson's black spot if ever there was one. Nick had driven us to the airport only a month or so before. I'm spooked: five deaths, two uncles now dying, and my old maw collapsing. All that and now I'm back to another round of busy take-days. There's no beds, the juniors are pissed off again, we seem to have no secretaries this week, and the IT is still shite.

I'm beginning to think enough is enough. But then *ArtReview* asks for another report from Berlin; a ray of relief.

20

LET GO

There's a tune from the early 1990s by an electronic duo called Spooky. The dance music has a pulsating bass beat, but there is something off-kilter about it. A sample from a track by the Pixies and an orchestral snippet of trilling flutes (Stravinsky?) accompanies an immersive wash of synthesised strings and a whispered voice that repeatedly, insistently, presses this message: *Let go.* The track comes to mind in my last year working as a doctor. Maybe it is time to let go.

I've been reading articles by David Oliver, columnist for the *BMJ* and clinical vice-president of the RCP. He retweets a report in *The Independent* on how creeping privatisation of healthcare is undermining the NHS. That day I'm angered after I get a text from a friend who has had to pay to see a gastroenterologist privately to get an endoscopy because this has been cancelled four times on the NHS. That whispered voice: *Let go.*

Did you know that NHS consultant job plans are not transparent? I'm told you can't find out how many hours another consultant in your own hospital works. Unfairness abounds. Consultants are not held to account for their movements, not monitored for where they actually are on any given day. *You have difficulty holding some people to account.*

Let go.

I'm in a field near the sea and I'm thinking about J. D. Salinger and Holden Caulfield and how Holden misinterprets the famous poem by Robert Burns. Holden wants to save the kids from falling off the cliffs. He wants to catch them. He is the catcher in the rye. This, it strikes me, is what doctors want to do too. It's what I wanted to do. Catch people before they fall. But you can't do that for ever: it might be time to catch yourself.

Let go.

An academic is knighted for his work on communicating with patients and I'm irrationally irritated. I don't know him and I'm sure he means well, I'm sure he deserves it. I bet his work is terrific. But have any of these specialists in communication actually broken bad news at midnight to a kid scared out their wits, a kid you want to catch before they fall off the cliff? Have they dealt with relatives angry about how their daughter has become unwell after chemotherapy? Chemotherapy prescribed by their oncologist. Now her bone marrow is failing, she's infected, she's septicaemic: it's gone midnight and she's under *your* care, not the oncologist's. Why?

Let go.

Why can't we get this new drug? It's a resource issue.

Let go.

I read somewhere that there are about ten consultants in endocrinology who work in one expensive part of London but only two in a northern town for a similar population base; a grotesque, long-standing iniquity replicated elsewhere. A widespread postcode lottery exists in British healthcare uncorrected by either of the main political parties.

Let go.

I've got an angry spot on my cheek and I'm up at 6 a.m. tomorrow to face another take-day with no beds and—

Let go.

Oh no. Here's that couple of wasters with nothing organically wrong with them rumbling up the road now to outpatients in their matching mobility scooters they somehow purloined from—

Let go.

Someone called Donna (a Christian, a mother) tweets: 'Outrageous that the NHS will be funding prophylactic anti-HIV drugs. Time to privatise the system. I don't pay taxes to enable gay men to lead hedonistic lifestyles.'

Let go.

I'm due to do a speech at a graduation ceremony: the booklet has me down as doing a 'welcome to the NHS'. The parents and the clean newly qualified faces look up at me expectantly. Just before going on stage, the Dean comes up to me and says: 'Don't go on about the NHS.'

Let go.

'There's no beds.'

Let go.

'There's no SHO this week.'

Let go.

'There's no registrar this week.'

Let go.

'The house officers are all away at induction.'

'The IT has gone down again.'

'I'm just back from annual leave so I don't know any of the patients.'

'There's no diabetes nurses to take any of the calls this week.'

'You will not get a pay rise this year or next year or the year after that.'

'There's a complaint.'

'The coroner is on the phone.'

'Your clinics you wanted cancelled when you are on leave have not been cancelled.'

'There's an extra five patients on your clinic this afternoon.'

'Can you do another appraisal for us this month?'

'Can you fill out another survey for us?'

'The Care Quality Commission is coming.'

'We've heard the CQC report might be bad.'

'Can I ask you to have a quick look at this ECG?'

'Can you come to the front desk quickly, someone has collapsed.'

'Look at this bruise: bloody vampires!'

'Where do they send it to? A black pudding factory?'

'I'm a proper doctor, you know, not like you. I'm a PhD.'

'All that money wasted on IVF. They should pay for it. Not the taxpayer.'

'I don't understand what you are saying: it's your accent, it's very thick, isn't it?'

'Aren't you ever going to go back to Glasgow?'

'We are on black alert. Can I ask you to do another ward round?'

'I know it's Friday afternoon, but can you do this weekend on call for us?'

'Your request has been rejected.'

'Yes, I saw my GP and I'm not a racist but...'

'Are you any relation to Dr Quinn, medicine woman?'

Let go.

ArtReview asks if I'd like to do a two-page illustrated spread on Warsaw. I'd like that. I'd like that a lot. It's time to chase just one rabbit.

NHS CHIEFS WARN THAT HOSPITALS IN ENGLAND ARE ON THE BRINK OF COLLAPSE

This is the headline in one of the newspapers four months after I've retired in 2016.

I'm surprised to see so many physically healthy people on the streets. I've got used to being around the unwell. But the number of vulnerable mentally ill people out and about shocks me. A lot are no longer cared for in hospitals. There seems to be a national indifference to their plight. And not just in the UK: over in Vancouver there were an enormous number of people wandering around in states of frank psychosis. This was the true face of 'care in the community'.

Homelessness is rampant, with many people begging on the streets of Brighton, London. I never saw that growing up in 1970s East Kilbride.

The elderly trudge home laden with their bags of groceries. Some look at me with scorn; I feel like a draft dodger. Their faces ask: Why aren't you at work, why aren't you at the front?

I visit a pub with a sign like the old CBGB's club in Manhattan: they play ancient tunes by the New York Dolls. I remember seeing them, or what was left of them, in a Berlin club called White Trash. I went with the widower of my old secretary. He could barely walk to the place, such was his deep depression. The band made him smile but only just. A couple of years later I meet his new girlfriend and a year on from then he's married again and happier.

Music, art, books. I listen to the radio a lot more now: Tuesday nights with Mickey Bradley on Radio Ulster. There's surfing Spotify too. I find a great book about *actual* surfing, William Finnegan's *Barbarian Days*, but I'm not tempted to give it a try. I'm happy enough watching them ride the unimpressive breakers off Brighton beach. A stack of yellow boards with a broad red stripe lies near the West Pier. They belong to the Brighton Surf Rescue team. I squint into the sun and sit listening to the percussive clank of sail rope against mast.

I head back over to Berlin. I'm eating outside and hear a car screech then a horrid thump. A cyclist has been hit. A crowd forms quickly; a passing medic is in attendance. Soon an ambulance comes wailing into view. I wonder if I should go over but then hear she is stable, she is being dealt with, she needs trauma specialists not a physician. And then, and only then, do I realise that my time as a physician is truly over. I'm not a practising doctor any more. Leave it to the professionals. I was a doctor, but I'm not now. I'm content. I'm 'happy'.

Happiness. Talk to the dying about happiness: they have some idea of what it meant, what it means. Palliative care physicians maintain that one of the commonest statements they hear from the dying is this: *I wish I hadn't worked for so long.*

I slow down. Read a bit more carefully; look at paintings in more detail. Spend as much time with my wife as I can. Time is running short.

I buy yet another book on Duchamp. When asked to describe himself, Duchamp would say that he was 'a breather'. You can only laugh at that and agree with him and take a few more breaths. Which reminds me of On Kawara's telegrams with their simple message: *I Am Still Alive.* Physicians get skilled at disappearing in an ego sense when conversing with patients; it's not about us. It's about *them.*

My father on his death bed: he stared at me with a glazed opiated look of surprise and odd contentment then said in a rush (no: he was warning me; this I now realise) that 'it all goes by so quickly'. *It?* He meant life, his life and my life. He thought that death (as Duchamp said) was something that only happened to others. But now it was coming for him and in time it will come for me. He died way too young. At fifty-five I thought I might have less than seven years left. I knew it was time to do something else.

Time. Now it was time to take time, to slow time, however foolish that might seem. Another great line I love is from a pop song by Paddy McAloon: *I want extra time to play, afternoons in the hay.* I want time to *be* again.

Being comes from my wife, my family, my friends, the music, art and literature that I love. Shakespeare must have said something about this, no doubt. Help me, Will!

I'm sitting at home ploughing through videos of the Shakespeare comedies the BBC made in the early 1980s. Old Pyke with his Hamlet knowledge would be proud of me. Shakespeare: now there *was* a fuckin' comedian. I'm watching the end of *Love's Labour's Lost* and what I hear rings true. What I hear sums up my life as Dr Quin, medicine man.

Lord Biron of Navarre is pledging his troth to the newly bereaved Queen of France: he asks her to 'impose some service on me for thy love'. The Queen knows that Biron is yet another joker 'replete with mocks' and so she sets him this challenge:

> To weed this wormwood from your fruitful brain,
> And therewithal to win me if you please,
> Without the which I am not to be won,
> You shall this twelvemonth term from day to day
> Visit the speechless sick and still converse

With groaning wretches; and your task shall be
With all the fierce endeavour of your wit
To enforce the pained impotent to smile.

Biron is incredulous: what a task is this! He pleads with her:

To move wild laughter in the throat of death?
It cannot be, it is impossible.
Mirth cannot move a soul in agony.

The Queen insists that this is the only way to 'choke a gibing spirit'
and Biron duly capitulates:

A twelvemonth? Well, befall what will befall,
I'll jest a twelvemonth in a hospital.

Like many others in the NHS I have jested in hospitals for more than
a twelvemonth. I jested and jibed in hospitals for thirty-three years.
Many go the full forty; some even more. Thirty-three multiplied by
twelvemonths, thirty-three twelvemonths with the speechless sick,
those 'deaf'd with the clamours of their own dear groans'. The sick
have heard enough of my idle scorns. Hopefully I made some of those
'pained impotent' smile. Hopefully. But I'm still not a fuckin' comedian.

After leaving I'm asked to write a piece for the *British Medical Journal* about the NHS and I give it the title 'Everything Must Go'. I
stuff as many Steely Dan quotations as I can into my polemic. More
pop quotation, more referential mania. The message is that we're
going out of business. The editors want something more upbeat,
they want concrete ideas on how we can save the NHS. They want

to cut all the Donald Fagen mentions, but I can't do that. I think Donald's diagnosis for America is ours too.

But some things *are* looking up. The current appraisal and revalidation process hopefully reduces mistakes and the clunking insensitivities of the past. There's always hope in medicine. Stem cells can now be turned into insulin-producing beta cells. Pretty soon there's hope that people with Type 1 diabetes might even be 'cured'. They will not need to inject themselves. They will pass me in the street maybe, like a lady I once referred for a pancreas transplant, and I'll wave to them and ask how they are getting on and they will beam and say: 'Great!' They'll say: 'I'm great because I don't need to see the likes of you *ever again!*'

I'm walking near the theatre in Brighton with my wife and suddenly someone rushes up to us. A woman our age, tall and slim with something of the refined southern English glamour you might associate with the Mitford sisters. She catches her breath and says: 'Dr Quin! How are you? You remember me, don't you?'

I do: she had a phaeochromocytoma. We diagnosed it, stuck her on the drugs, got the surgeons to take it out. The tumour dropped in my gloved palm like a gift. You don't get to cure that many people and I smile in recognition when she laughs and says: 'You *do* remember me!'

As she stands amongst the passing shoppers she is profuse in her thanks then leans forward and kisses me on the cheek when she hears I've retired: 'Have a lovely time and you take care of yourself!'

We part but seconds later she runs back to us and is now stroking my wife's arm: 'I hope you don't mind me doing that? Kissing him. I didn't mean it... you know, *that way*. I just mean, well... he saved my life. And for that I'm eternally grateful.'

What a great job I had. Some doctors who have quit the profession say that they would never recommend it, that kids should pick something else, that they should give medical school a miss. I disagree. If you're a young person reading this thinking of doing medicine: do it. We need you.

My wife nods and laughs and then we watch the woman turn away towards the Pavilion. I'm now definitive that a chunk of my life has now finished, that it is time to start afresh. We walk together down to the sea and look at the waves crashing in towards us.

EPILOGUE

And now it's April 2020. You know what has happened. I'm temporarily re-registered with the GMC; I've filled in the forms for HR; I'm signed up again with my defence union; I've bought a new book on evidence-based endocrinology.

I'm down to do my first clinic in four years next week.

ACKNOWLEDGEMENTS

In memory of my dad, John, and William Robertson.

Many thanks to Chris Paling and Martin Herbert for all their encouragement and teaching on writing.

I've been very lucky to work with an army of fantastic doctors, nurses and secretaries down through the years and I salute them all, in particular those who trained me referred to in the text: you know who you are. Those working in the NHS right now are truly heroic people given the impact of the Covid-19 virus. The many deaths of staff are a tragedy and a scandal that awaits proper scrutiny.

Thanks to my agent Kevin Pocklington for keeping the faith and my editor Olivia Beattie for her advice and eyes as focused as an electron microscope. I've also had fantastic advice on writing from Mark Rappolt, David Terrien, JJ Charlesworth, Oliver Basciano, Louise Darblay, Robert Barry, Rüdiger Shafer and Jacayln Carley. And thanks for welcome comments on the stories and the text to David Marshall, Miles Fisher, Pavel Dominik, Ian Scobie and Hilda McMillan. I'm very grateful to Stephen Gallacher for telling me to get that spot on my arm sorted.

My mum, brothers, sister and all my friends have put up with hearing various versions of these stories over the years and I thank them for their patience, love and affection.

Lastly but most importantly I want to thank my wife Maureen, my own lucky star, for all her love and being.